D0074825

LOST WORDS

LOST WORDS

NARRATIVES OF LANGUAGE
AND THE BRAIN,
1825–1926

L. S. Jacyna

PRINCETON UNIVERSITY PRESS

PRINCETON AND OXFORD

LIBRARY OF CONGRESS CATALOGING-IN-PUBLICATION DATA

JACYNA, L. S.

LOST WORDS : NARRATIVES OF LANGUAGE

AND THE BRAIN, 1825–1926 / L. S. JACYNA.

P.   CM.

INCLUDES BIBLIOGRAPHICAL REFERENCES AND INDEX.

ISBN 0-691-00413-7 (CL : ALK. PAPER)

1. APHASIA—HISTORY. I. TITLE

RC425.J33   2000

616.85′52′009—dc21   99-089724

CONTENTS

ILLUSTRATIONS

ACKNOWLEDGMENTS

I WROTE THIS book while holding a Senior Research Fellowship awarded by the Wellcome Trust. I wish to acknowledge the Trust's generous support of my work. Thanks are due to the staff of the Library of the Wellcome Institute for the History of Medicine who did much to facilitate the research involved in the project. Chris Lawrence, Paul Lerner, and Roy Porter read various portions of the manuscript in draft and offered valuable criticisms, as did two anonymous readers. I have also benefited from the comments of seminar audiences at the Wellcome Institute for the History of Medicine, the Science Studies Unit, Edinburgh, John Hopkins University, Princeton, and the University of California, San Francisco. Emily Wilkinson and Sam Elworthy provided support and encouragement during the production process. An earlier version of chapter 1 appeared as "Construing Silence: Narratives of Language Loss in Early Nineteenth-Century France," *Journal of the History of Medicine* 49 (1994): 333–61.

LOST WORDS

INTRODUCTION

THIS BOOK is a series of readings in a body of medical literature. The second half of the nineteenth century saw the emergence of a new genre of writing dealing with the relations between language and the human brain;[1] during this period a new condition known as "aphasia" emerged as an object of intense investigation. As a study of the writing by nineteenth- and twentieth-century doctors about this topic, *Lost Words* is a contribution to the history of a medical specialty; research into aphasia was central to the generation of an intellectual identity for neurology. The book is also relevant to wider issues of the relation of patient and practitioner in modern Western societies. Because aphasia studies were indispensable to any attempt to localize language in the cerebral cortex, it necessarily touches on major themes in the history of what are now known as the neurosciences. The subject matter of *Lost Words* is, moreover, relevant to current concerns with the cultural history of the self: it describes a moment when crucial aspects of personality were shown to be dependent on material organization.

It is possible to assign an inception date to the literature on aphasia: 1861. As soon as this date is proposed, however, a variety of alternative starting points occur. While I am of the view that the 1860s *are* the decisive decade in initiating the literature with which this book deals, the study begins by considering a number of earlier texts. One of these (that of Bouillaud) was retrospectively awarded a status within the corpus of aphasia studies. More important, it already displays some of the necessary preconditions for what might be called mature aphasiology.

While the literature of aphasia possesses a starting point—or rather several more or less plausible beginnings—it has no terminus. Aphasiology is very much an ongoing enterprise as the most casual survey of current medical bibliographies will reveal. The decision to conclude this study in 1926 with Henry Head's *Aphasia and Kindred Disorders* is therefore to some extent, though not entirely, arbitrary.

The book does not pretend to be a comprehensive survey of the literature of aphasia between 1825 and 1926. Instead it takes certain texts from that literature—some of them "classics," others more obscure—and subjects them to a variety of readings. The expression "medical literature" is

---

[1] For useful collections of some of the major texts in this literature see: H. Hecaen and J. Dubois, *La naissance de la neuropsychologie du langage 1825–1865* (Paris: Flammarion, 1969); Paul Eling, *Reader in the History of Aphasia: From [Franz] Gall to [Norman] Geschwind* (Amsterdam: Benjamins, 1994).

therefore used here in a more deliberate way than is usual to refer to a body of medical writing that bears sustained critical scrutiny. The texts in question have been chosen less with the aim of identifying key moments in the development of the modern understanding of the relation of language to the brain than in order to illuminate certain definitive aspects of this body of literature. I am, moreover, also anxious to demonstrate the possibilities of certain strategies for the reading of medical texts. I believe that these ways of reading have an applicability that goes beyond the subject matter of the present study.

My emphasis is on the texts themselves rather than on their authors.[2] I maintain that in important respects the signification of these documents cannot be referred to the motives or impulses of the individuals producing them. The primary aim of the book is not therefore to provide intellectual biographies of the authors of these writings. Thus, although I discuss Paul Broca's early contribution to the literature at some length, that discussion is not about "Broca" as such: that is a name conventionally assigned the authorship of a collection of texts some of which are relevant to this study. In the case of the debate at the Société d'Anthropologie upon which I focus, moreover, Broca's utterances form part of a composite text in which there are other participating voices.

To a still more marked degree chapter 3 has no protagonist. It seeks to show the order, the conditions of coherence, underlying a representative selection of texts drawn from what can be called the classic period of nineteenth-century aphasiology. When I cite a text by, for example, Carl Wernicke, it is with this end in mind. To object that other texts by that author—or even the *same* text—can with some plausibility be cited in different contexts is beside the point.

Even when a particular author, John Hughlings Jackson or Henry Head, is at the center of a chapter, it is the writings ascribed to that name that provide the focus of attention. The aim in these cases is not to show how a particular text is determined by the supposed intentions of an author, nor to show its place within his overall literary output. It is rather to demonstrate how these classic aphasiological texts can be read in novel ways to show within them the presence of unexpected contingencies. It is also to insist that a scientific text is not a transparent window upon reality but itself a dense object of study.[3]

---

[2] For an excellent discussion of the various forms of concern with linguistic questions in recent historiography see: Penelope J. Corfield, "Introduction: Historians and Language," in idem (ed.), *Language, History and Class* (Oxford: Blackwell, 1991), pp. 1–29.

[3] For a review of the growing awareness in the history of science of the need for close attention to language see: J. V. Golinski, "Language, Discourse and Science," in R. C. Olby, G. N. Cantor, J. R. R. Christie, and M. J. S. Hodge, *Companion to the History of Science* (London: Routledge, 1989), pp. 110–123; L. J. Jordanova, "Introduction," to idem (ed.),

I recognize that by adopting this approach I leave myself open to various criticisms—perhaps the most serious of which is that such concentration on the text is merely a new species of idealism. What has already been said is at least a partial answer to this reproach: texts figure in this book not as the expression of the thoughts of a few great men or even of several smaller ones. Still less are they seen as the incidental expressions of a pure, transcendent natural knowledge. The emphasis is much more upon the way in which every author must write in a language of which he or she is not fully the master; discourse exists as a datum which conditions and exceeds all efforts at individual expression.

Texts must, moreover, be understood as the products of concrete historical processes;[4] in some cases, indeed, these documents are the *only* relics of that history. As one historian has remarked, "the relationships constituting hospital medicine were both made, and made visible, primarily when those involved in it wrote about them."[5] chapter 3, in particular, seeks to depict the production of these scientific texts as a species of work dependent on a range of prior and parallel activities; and, in our culture, work is conventionally regarded as an embodied, material process.[6]

I am, above all, acutely aware that at the center of these processes were damaged and diseased bodies; we can, however, only know anything about those suffering individuals through the webs of language that were woven around their afflictions. (It may even be argued that these bodies together

---

Languages of Nature: Critical Essays on Science and Literature (London: Free Association, 1986), pp. 15–47. The role of texts in generating, as opposed to merely communicating, knowledge is found in Steven Shapin, "Pump and Circumstance: Robert Boyle's Literary Technology," *Social Studies of Science* 14 (1984): 481–520; Steven Shapin and Simon Schaffer, *Leviathan and the Air-Pump: Hobbes, Boyle, and the Experimental Method* (Princeton: Princeton University Press, 1985), esp. pp. 60–69. Other studies in the history of science sensitive to linguistic issues include: Evelyn Fox Keller, *Secrets of Life and Death: Essays on Language, Gender and Science* (New York: Routledge, 1992); Donna Haraway, *Primate Visions: Gender, Race, and Nature in the World of Modern Science* (London: Routledge, 1989); Marco Beretta, "The Grammar of Matter: Chemical Nomenclature during the 18th Century," in Roger Chartier and Pietro Corsi (eds.), *Sciences et langues en Europe* (Paris: Centre Alexandre Koyré, 1996), pp. 109–125.

[4] For a perceptive account of how an emphasis upon symbolic resources—linguistic and otherwise—is fully compatible with a historical materialism see: Raphael Samuel, "Reading the Signs," *History Workshop* 31–32 (1991): 88–109, especially pp. 104–5.

[5] Susan C. Lawrence, *Charitable Knowledge: Hospital Pupils and Practitioners in Eighteenth-Century London* (Cambridge: Cambridge University Press, 1996), p. 23. For an example of how new ways of writing formed an integral part of the development of innovatory medical practices see: Jacalyn Duffin, *To See with a Better Eye: A Life of R. T. H. Laennec* (Princeton: Princeton University Press, 1998), p. 141.

[6] This is incidentally to discount the notion that the generation of knowledge is an immaterial, transcendent process. These dichotomies are considered in Christopher Lawrence and Steven Shapin, *Science Incarnate: Historical Embodiments of Natural Knowledge* (Chicago: University of Chicago Press, 1998), especially p. 4.

with their afflictions exist *because* of these discursive practices.[7]) Foucault's remarks about the literary aspect of the disciplinary process are equally applicable to the work of the clinic:

> The examination leaves behind it a whole meticulous archive constituted in terms of bodies and days. The examination that places individuals in a field of surveillance also situates them in a network of writing; it engages them in a whole mass of documents that capture and fix them. . . . A 'power of writing' was constituted as an essential part in the mechanisms of discipline.[8]

If the book has a protagonist it is the "aphasic," an entity that emerged in the pages of medical journals and monographs in the latter part of the nineteenth century. The afflicted men and women who supplied the raw material for this invention mostly survive only as the objects of this discourse. The "lost words" of the title refers not only to their physical disabilities but also to their lack of power to influence the acts of representation within which they were entwined. Where exceptions to this rule occur they do so for particular reasons.

A number of firsthand accounts of the experience of aphasia from the period covered by this book do exist; one of these is discussed in chapter 1. It would, however, be a mistake to imagine that these narratives constitute a more natural or authentic account of the condition; they do provide a contrasting set of representations that help demonstrate the partiality and contingency of a ruling discourse. "Experience," whether of work, illness, or any other mode of life, is never raw.[9]

But it is only more recently that a literary form has arisen that gives the speechless[10] man and woman the opportunity to record his or her own account of their affliction. Notably, a number of moving descriptions of the experience of aphasia appeared in a collection published in 1992. One sufferer recalled: "I was in a different world really. . . . It was like being on

---

[7] For an exposition of this extreme Foucauldian antihumanist position see: David Armstrong, "Bodies of Knowledge/Knowledge of Bodies," in Colin Jones and Roy Porter (eds.), *Reassessing Foucault: Power, Medicine and the Body* (London: Routledge, 1994), 17–27, pp. 21–22.

[8] Michel Foucault, *Discipline and Punish: The Birth of the Prison*, translated by Alan Sheridan, (Harmondsworth: Penguin, 1977), p. 189. For an account of the development of record making as an integral aspect of neurological work see: Christopher G. Goetz, Michael Bonduelle, and Toby Gelfand, *Charcot: Constructing Neurology* (Oxford: Oxford University Press, 1995), pp. 67–68.

[9] See the remarks in: Patrick Joyce, *Democratic Subjects: The Self and the Social in Nineteenth-Century England* (Cambridge: Cambridge University Press, 1994), pp. 4–5.

[10] I use this term to refer loosely to the full gamut of language disorders derived from injury to the brain. In fact, few sufferers are altogether deprived of speech, and various aspects of language other than speech can also be affected.

another planet." Another described "a terrible feeling of being encapsulated in a black bottomless pit. . . . [I]t was as though my net of words had been ostracized and banned to another unknown recess of my mind." A third was more pithy: "I seemed to have become an idiot."[11] These quotations provide striking evidence of the importance of a mastery of language to the sense of self.

The "aphasic" that emerged in the course of the later nineteenth century can thus be considered both as the object of a clinical-scientific gaze and as the product of an extensive work process. We can identify various aspects of this process. It included the verbal and physical examination of patients and the dissection of cadavers along with the incidental preparation of pathological specimens. But (with the exception of some surviving museum artifacts) we only know these things through the medium of the literary aspect of aphasiological work; all these other operations were preliminary to the generation of texts.[12] The "facts" of aphasiology attained their final form as written statements available to a community of readers. One of the goals of this study is to explore the ways in which the structure of these documents creates certain forms of heuristic possibility while eliding others.[13]

The aphasic who, in all his particularity and partiality, inhabits these texts is necessarily a fragmentary being. That partiality is in important respects a matter of gender: I will argue that the aphasic is conceived as an impaired *man* regardless of the sex of the patient—hence my use of the masculine pronoun to describe him. He is the speechless person seen from a determinate point of view—a viewpoint endowed with the power to ensure its exclusivity: "Every idea originates through equating the un-

---

[11] Gill Edelman and Robert Greenwood, *Jumbly Words, and Rights Where Wrongs Should Be: The Experience of Aphasia from the Inside* (Kibworth: Far Communications, 1992), pp. 83, 98–99, 119. For other firsthand narratives see: David Knox, *Portrait of Aphasia* (Detroit: Wayne State University Press, 1971); Helen Harlan Wulf, *Aphasia, My World Alone* (Detroit: Wayne State University Press, 1979). A more recent collection makes the assumption that the recollections of physicians and neuroscientists who have themselves suffered from some neurological condition are of special value: Narinder Kapur, *Injured Brains of Medical Minds: Views from Within* (Oxford: Oxford University Press, 1997). See pp. 49–116 for firsthand accounts of aphasia. It is notable that these narratives are not allowed to speak for themselves; an editorial "commentary" is appended to each patient's account.

[12] On the role of narrative construction in medical work see: Kathryn Montgomery Hunter, *Doctor's Stories: The Narrative Structure of Medical Knowledge* (Princeton: Princeton University Press, 1991). Bruno Latour and Steve Woolgar, *Laboratory Life: The Social Construction of Scientific Facts* (Beverly Hills: Sage, 1979) stresses the central importance of documents in the everyday life of modern laboratory science; see especially pp. 52–53.

[13] On how narrative structures shape medical investigation see: Allan Young, *The Harmony of Illusions: Inventing Post-Traumatic Stress Disorder* (Princeton: Princeton University Press, 1995), pp. 169–70, 190.

equal."[14] These inequalities, if recognized at all, are dismissed as irrelevant to the task in hand. The individual case matters only in so far as it serves to help build "a pyramidal order with castes and grades, to create a new world of laws, privileges, sub-orders, [and] delimitations."[15]

The partiality of a discourse is manifested in its ruling metaphors.[16] Sometimes these metaphors are manifest and clearly distinguished from the nonfigurative parts of a text. Thus when Jean-Baptiste Bouillaud writes of the "great cerebral university, corresponding to this grand university in which are comprised all the sciences, all the arts," he is making overt use of a rhetorical figure in the context of a more strictly scientific account of the brain couched in more prosaic language.[17]

However, such examples give an inadequate impression of the operations of metaphor in scientific texts.[18] Later in the same discourse Bouillaud describes language as one of the most elevated among "the fundamental faculties . . . which by their concourse, their fraternal association, and, if I may say so, their holy alliance, constitute the complete system, the general body and UNITY [*faisceau général et UN*] of our mind [*entendement*]."[19] In this instance is the use of "faculty" still a metaphoric allusion to the constitution of a university or to be taken as a literal reference to a particular theory of the constitution of mind?[20]

Close reading reveals that metaphor pervades even the most overtly literal forms of writing; the most powerful metaphors are those no longer recognized as such.[21] Nietzsche again provides a valuable point of refer-

---

[14] Friedrich Nietzsche, "On Truth and Falsity in their Ultramodern Sense," in *The Complete Works of Friedrich Nietzsche*, edited by Oscar Levy, vol. 2 (London: T. N. Foulis, 1911), p. 179.

[15] Ibid.

[16] I pass over the various other social processes by which any particular view of reality is established as the basis for a program of research. For some suggestive comments see: Young, *Harmony of Illusions*, pp. 102–3, 121–24.

[17] Jean-Baptiste Bouillaud, "Discussion sur la faculté du langage articulé," *Bullétin de l'Académie Impériale de Médecine* 30 (1864–65): 575–638, on p. 594.

[18] For extended discussions of the instability of the distinctions between figurative and referential language in scientific texts see: Andrew E. Benjamin, Geoffrey N. Cantor, and John R. R. Christie (eds.), *The Figural and the Literal: Problems of Language in the History of Science and Philosophy, 1630–1800* (Manchester: Manchester University Press, 1987).

[19] Bouillaud, "Discussion," p. 605. For a general discussion of metaphor in the history of psychology and the neurosciences see: John C. Marshall, "Minds, Machines and Metaphors," *Social Studies of Science* 7 (1977): 475–488.

[20] I forgo the opportunity to tease out the many other interesting features of this passage. What are we, for instance, to make of the phrase "holy alliance," an apparent allusion to a political configuration from the recent past that was repugnant to Bouillaud's party?

[21] Richard Rorty has, for instance, shown how the whole of Western metaphysics rest on a suppressed metaphor, namely, the supposed analogy between knowledge and perception: *Philosophy and the Mirror of Nature* (Oxford: Blackwell, 1980), pp. 159–63.

ence. He pointed out how, for instance, the supposed "mechanism" of auditory perception was tacitly figural: "A nerve-stimulus; first transformed into a percept! First metaphor! The percept again copied into a sound! Second metaphor!"[22] One of the aims of this book is to draw attention to some of the constitutive but effectively invisible metaphors that permeate discourse about language and the brain.[23]

While the construction of the aphasic is primarily of significance as an addition to the burgeoning of a neurological literature in the later nineteenth century, it possesses a wider cultural relevance. It was, in the first place, dependent on the conjunction of events earlier in the nineteenth century that Foucault calls the "Birth of the Clinic."[24] This development produced a material and epistemological machinery that made patients and their pathologies available for novel forms of medical productivity. Hospital patients whose treatment was seen more as a privilege than as a right were, in particular, adapted to these purposes. The literary forms of aphasiology—the case history and the autopsy report—are the typical tools of all hospital medicine.

Because of their peculiar subject matter, however, this literature also possesses unique dimensions. They deal with what came to be known (in a telling phrase) as the diseases of the "higher," most distinctively *human*, functions of the brain. The aphasiological text therefore also possesses an anthropological import: it constitutes a moment in the emergence of a natural science of man.[25] The ability to speak and use language in other ways was of special importance in defining humanity; indeed, the ability to speak was often deemed *the* defining characteristic of man, the character that distinguished him from the mere brute. There was, in particular, a close association between language, thought, and individual liberty. Through language—and above all through speech[26]—the human essence represented itself to its fellows, to those capable of recognizing such utter-

[22] Nietzsche, "On Truth," p. 178.

[23] It is worth noting in passing that the linguist, Roman Jakobson, used the figure of the metaphor, and of the contrasting trope of metonymy, in his efforts to arrive at a classification of the language deficits characteristic of different forms of aphasia: "Two Aspects of Language and Two Types of Aphasic Disturbance," in *Selected Writings*, vol. 2 (The Hague: Mouton, 1971), pp. 239–59.

[24] Michel Foucault, *The Birth of the Clinic: An Archaeology of Medical Perception*, trans. A. M. Sheridan Smith (New York: Pantheon Books, 1975).

[25] I am of course aware of the exclusions involved in the assumption that "man" represented the whole of humanity. On this partiality of vision see: Ornella Moscucci, *The Science of Woman: Gynaecology and Gender in England 1800–1929* (Cambridge: Cambridge University Press, 1990), pp. 31–32. The aphasic is to be considered as a damaged version of this distinctly masculine construct.

[26] See the remarks on "phonocentrism" in Jacques Derrida, *Of Grammatology* (Baltimore: Johns Hopkins Press, 1976), pp. 11–12.

ances for what they were, tokens of a deliberative and determining person.[27] Witness, for example, the importance attached to the right of free speech in liberal democratic systems.

Within this framework the aphasic was a peculiarly portentous being. Because of the impairment of his ability to utter and comprehend words, he attained a liminal status; his human identity was open to question: "Nothing deserves the name of man except what is able to speak."[28] Rather than being a sovereign individual in command of his organs, his body seemed to overpower efforts at self-expression.[29] These links between language, humanity, and mental presence do much to explain the fascination of the aphasiological project.

The aphasic was portentous not only, however, on account of the nature of his impairment but also because of what he revealed about the conditions for the healthy exercise of man's defining characteristic. The literature of aphasia established an intimacy and dependence between what had been regarded as a uniquely spiritual faculty and man's corporeal part. Aphasia showed that language possessed a bodily organ—or, perhaps more to the point, that a material organ possessed *it*. Language was, in other words, endowed with the status of a function; it was part of the proper domain of biological science.

The discovery of aphasia thus formed part of a larger movement, one in which "Man's finitude is heralded."[30] The nineteenth century was an epoch when what had been formerly deemed transcendent faculties of perception and cognition were found to have anatomico-physiological conditions; the positive contents of biological sciences demonstrated the necessary limitations of human knowledge.[31] The case of aphasia revealed that

---

[27] A contemporary statement of this vision of the centrality of language and of the profound and far-reaching consequences for the individual when it is damaged is found in the definition provided by the American National Institute on Deafness and Other Communication Disorders: "Language is the expression of human communication through which knowledge, belief and behavior can be experienced, explained and shared. The ability to manipulate language to satisfy needs and desires and to express thoughts, observations and values is an important human pursuit that directly infuences the quality of life for any individual. Language impairments impede social development, academic performance, employment opportunities and economic self-sufficiency." http://www.nih.gov/nidcd/language.htm

[28] Max Müller, "Lectures on Mr Darwin's Philosophy of Language. Second Lecture," *Fraser's Magazine* 7 (1873): 659–78, on pp. 666–67.

[29] See the suggestive comments in: Derek Attridge, *Peculiar Language: Literature as Difference from the Renaissance to James Joyce* (London: Methuen, 1988), pp. 160–62.

[30] Michel Foucault, *The Order of Things: An Archaeology of the Human Sciences* (London: Routledge, 1974), p. 313.

[31] On the corporealization of vision during this period see: Jonathan Crary, *Techniques of the Observer: On Vision and Modernity in the Nineteenth Century* (Cambridge, Mass.: MIT Press, 1990), especially pp. 70–71, 79–81.

there was a *nature* to language, a faculty previously associated with the immaterial part of man abutting on a supernal realm.

The existence of a bodily mechanism for the execution of linguistic performances had, of course, been recognized long before. What changed in the nineteenth century was that such structures as the tongue and larynx were now revealed as strictly secondary, surface organs. The primary organs of language resided in the uncharted territories of the brain. There was, in short, a secret to language that only a particular medical-scientific endeavor could unravel. The aphasiological project was the self-conscious response to this novel problematic.

Alluding in *The Order of Things* to some of the products of this enterprise, Michel Foucault drew a distinction between this biological assault upon the seat of language and the linguistic studies proper to the "human sciences" that had commenced about the same time. He insisted that

> the anatomy of the cortical centres of language, cannot in any way be considered as sciences of man. This is because the object of those sciences is never posited in the mode of being of a biological function . . . ; it is rather its reverse, or the hollow it would leave; it begins at the point, not where the action or the effects stop, but where that function's own being stops—at that point where representations are set free . . . ; research into the intracortical connections between the different centres of linguistic integration (auditive, visual, motor) is not the province of the human sciences.[32]

Foucault here indicates the conventional distinction between the social and the biological sciences. Man is a proper object of study in both fields; but while the latter delineate his material nature, the former are concerned with his cultural activity. In the one man is a passive object shaped by forces undetermined by the array of representations available to him; in the other he is an active agent who, within limits, makes his own destiny.

The discovery of the aphasic had, however, implications that threaten to overwhelm this agreeable division of labour. Aphasiology shows that the most basic of man's representational powers—the ability to form concepts and to employ words—is rooted in his material nature. All dichotomies between the cultural and the biological are therefore at most provisional or tendentious. The chapter in the history of science with which this book deals thus constitutes an episode of some moment in the emergence of a comprehensive scientific naturalism. The demonstration that language too was a function of man's animal part brought it within the domain of the natural sciences; it was no longer the sole preserve of *Geisteswissenschaft*.[33]

---

[32] Foucault, *Order*, p. 352.

[33] This encroachment of natural science on the territory of the humanities provoked particular resistance in Germany; the issue came to a head in a 1874 debate on aphasia at the

The Historiography of Aphasia

The writing of the history of aphasia began at virtually the same time as the invention of the concept. A number of interconnected threads can be distinguished within this literature. There was, on the one hand, a paradoxical attempt to deny the historicity of the condition. Because the aphasic was deemed to be a natural object he should occur in all periods and in all cultures—wherever man existed as a language user. Thus old texts were scoured for instances of aphasia before the name: this quest of course encompassed medical texts, beginning with the works of Hippocrates and extending to more recent sources such as the writings of William Cullen, the two Franks, and Phillipe Pinel. All of these writers had, it was claimed, recorded conditions which could in retrospect be identified as of aphasia.

More obscure authors could also yield similar anticipations. In a 1950 article Wladimir Eliasberg questioned Walther Riese's claim that after 1861 "the problems involved in aphasia appeared in their totality with almost explosive suddenness."[34] Eliasberg cited an eighteenth-century account of a case of language loss to show that these issues had been aired at an earlier date. He had no doubt that the disorder in question had been one "which we today would describe as a combination of subcortical motor aphasia with conduction aphasia." The contemporary attempts to explain the case were, however, inadequate because "Those early psychologists relied on too few, too casual, and too superficial observations."[35]

The search was, moreover, not confined to medical works; a much wider range of sources, including the Bible and classical texts, were also mined to provide further instances of the presence throughout time of the imperfectly recognized aphasic. William A. Hammond claimed that "The fact that the faculty of speech may be deranged independently either of the will, paralysis, or loss of voice, appears to have been noticed at a very early period in the progress of science." He proceeded to corroborate the point by citing a miscellaneous collection of texts—beginning with the Book of Isaiah.[36]

Berlin Anthropological Society. See: Michael Hagner, "Aspects of Brain Localization in Late XIXth Century Germany," in Claude Debru, *Essays in the History of the Physiological Sciences*, Clio Medica 33 (Amsterdam: 1995), pp. 73–88; idem, *Homo Cerebralis: Der Wandel vom Seelenorgan zum Gehirn* (Berlin: Berlin Verlag, 1997), pp. 279–93.

[34] W. G. Eliasberg, "A Contribution to the Prehistory of Aphasia," *Journal of the History of Medicine* 5 (1950): 96–101, p. 96.

[35] Ibid., pp. 99, 100.

[36] William A. Hammond, *A Treatise on the Diseases of the Nervous System*, 8th ed., (New York: D. Appleton, 1886), p. 183.

Another thread in the historiography of aphasia was more rigorous and more purposeful than this species of antiquarianism. While it did not deny the natural status of the aphasic, this tradition shifted the emphasis to establishing which authors had first adequately represented the existence of this entity. The point of the history now became to determine what *credit* belonged to the various individuals who had contributed to the emergent discourse of aphasia.

This variety of historiography tended to a more saltatory—almost catastrophic—view of the relation between past and present. Speaking at a meeting of the Académie Impériale de Médecine in 1865, Armand Trousseau poured scorn on those who scoured old case histories for instances of what might now be called aphasia, but at the time had been described as "alalia," or dumbness. He declared that "Sauvages [and] Cullen have written the most deplorable things about alalia. Monstrous clinical and physiological errors occur." Likewise, although the "erudite" Joseph Frank had described many cases of alalia he had not distinguished any facts that were pathognomonic of aphasia; it was clear that "he had not known how to make the distinction."[37]

In the clinical lectures he delivered at the Hôtel-Dieu of Paris, Trousseau was more specific about what constituted the inadequacy of premodern observations of speech loss: they failed to address the crucial question of the cerebral localization of the linguistic faculties.[38] This was a task reserved for the moderns. He then turned to the task of specifying the particular achievements of those individuals who had—or were alleged to have—contributed in one way or another to seminal investigations in the field of language and the brain.

During the early days of the discourse these discussions tended to revolve around relatively few names. There was much dispute about whether Franz Josef Gall, the originator of the doctrine that each psychological faculty possessed its special organ in the cerebrum,[39] should be accorded a place in the genealogy of modern notions of the subject on the grounds of his identification of a "seat" for the faculty of language in the anterior portions of the brain. The general view was that although Gall was eventually proved to be correct, this was something of a lucky guess; he was right for the wrong reasons. Jean-Baptise Bouillaud's contribution (see chapter 1) was somewhat less difficult to acknowledge and evaluate. He was an avowed follower of Gall; but while his master had based his localization

[37] A. Trousseau, "Sur la faculté du langage articulé," *Bullétin de l'Académie Impériale de Médecine* 30 (1864–65): 659–675, on pp. 660–661.

[38] A. Trousseau, *Clinique médicale de l'Hôtel-Dieu de Paris* (Paris: Baillière, 1865), p. 593.

[39] On Gall's "organology" see: Edwin Clarke and L. S. Jacyna, *Nineteenth-Century Origins of Neuroscientific Concepts* (Berkeley: University of California Press, 1987), pp. 220–44.

upon spurious anecdotal evidence, Bouillaud proceeded upon the sound principles of the clinico-pathological method.

But by far the most important issue addressed in these debates was the significance to be assigned to the contributions made by Paul Broca in the 1860s to a scientific understanding of the relations between the faculty of articulate language and certain portions of the cerebral hemispheres. Broca's place in the genealogy of aphasia was for a time controversial: the originality of his observations was in particular challenged by Dax *père* and *fils*.[40] By c.1870, however, Broca had attained a secure status within the historiography of aphasia studies. Indeed it was generally conceded that his work *inaugurated* the modern era in the understanding of the relations between language and the brain. Broca thus acquired the status of the founding father of true aphasia studies. There was clearly a felt need for some such paternal presence in this as in other branches of science.

Bouillaud already adumbrated this view in 1865 when he wrote of the dawn of a "new era" in the aftermath of Broca's conversion to the doctrine of the localization of the faculty of language in the brain.[41] But Bouillaud maintained that Broca's efforts were part of a larger "movement" in medicine rather than as merely the achievement of an individual. He was especially anxious to uphold his own claims and those of his son-in-law Simon Alexandre Ernest Auburtin to have contributed as least as much to the localizationist enterprise. The secular tendency was, however, to demote Bouillaud and his like to the status of precursors who had approximated to an insight that Broca alone had fully attained.

Thus in an 1884 discussion of researches and speculations on language and the brain, Charles Féré insisted, after reviewing various of these precursors, that:

> It is Broca (1861) who first conjoined a good clinical observation to a proper autopsy; it is he who first related the loss of articulate language, motor aphasia precisely defined, to a lesion accurately localized in a defined area of the cerebral cortex, in the posterior part of the third frontal convolution. . . . No doubt one can go back to Hippocrates . . . [for] the first observation of impaired language; but it is not enough to observe, it is necessary to comprehend.

---

[40] This particular contest has received a good deal of attention. See: Francis Schiller, *Paul Broca: Founder of French Anthropology, Explorer of the Brain* (Berkeley: University of California Press, 1979), pp. 193–97; Daniel Roe and Stanley Finger, "Gustave Dax and his Fight for Recognition: An Overlooked Chapter in the Early History of Cerebral Dominance," *Journal of the History of the Neurosciences*, 1996, 5: 228–40.

[41] Jean-Baptiste Bouillaud, "Sur la faculté du langage articulé," *Bullétin de l'Académie Impériale de Médecine* 30 (1864–65): 584.

In other words, Broca's contribution was valid because it conformed to what was deemed the correct literary form. To reinforce the point Féré drew an analogy between aphasia and hysteria. If "two centuries ago a magistrate's clerk described the contortions of a convulsive, which we today recognise as the classic episodes of an hysterical seizure, are we to say that he understood and described hystero-epilepsy?"[42] Before an affliction could be given its right name, the conditions for its understanding and representation had first to exist.

Some years earlier Carl Wernicke had made much the same point more succinctly. In the preamble to his own classic aphasiological text Wernicke announced that

> I shall pass over the host of older works regarding this problem . . . and shall turn immediately to Broca. This author was first to reject broad, indefinite expanses of the cortex as sites of speech areas and instead ventured to designate a very circumscribed, anatomically-specific region as the seat of this function.[43]

Here the particularity of Broca's achievement is specified more closely; it lay in the fact that he provided localization of a certain kind: one that conformed to Wernicke's standards of scientific precision.

By the end of the nineteenth century Broca's once controversial writings on the seat of language had attained a monumental standing. They constituted an originating text for the discourse of aphasia. This near sacred status goes far to explain why Pierre Marie's attack early in the twentieth century upon what had become Broca's dogma was deemed so shocking a piece of iconoclasm (see chapter 6).

Broca therefore possessed a unique status in the history of aphasia; he stood as a patriarchal figure who had engendered all the writing on the subject that followed. With time, however, other towering individuals emerged whose contribution to the development of the discourse was deemed almost as significant. When in 1888 M. Allen Starr attempted to

---

[42] Charles Féré, "Des troubles de l'usage des signes," *Revue philosophique* 17 (1884): 593–606, on pp. 595–596. For a similar vindication of Broca's claims against the pretensions of others (including Bouillaud) see: Désiré Bernard, *De l'aphasie et de ses diverses formes* (Paris: Lecrosnier et Babé, 1889), pp. 8–9. Féré's analogy between aphasia and the emergence of a scientific understanding of the symptoms of hysteria had extensive implications. For the cultural and political import of hysteria studies in late nineteenth-century France see: Jan Goldstein, *Console and Classify: The French Psychiatric Profession in the Nineteenth Century* (Cambridge: Cambridge University Press, 1987), pp. 371–74.

[43] Carl Wernicke, "The Aphasia Symptom Complex: A Psychological Study on an Anatomical Basis," in Gertrude H. Eggert (ed.), *Wernicke's Works on Aphasia: A Sourcebook and Review* (The Hague: Mouton, 1977), p. 100.

identify the most important moments in the growth of knowledge "regarding disturbances of speech and their important bearing upon the theory of localization of cerebral functions," he concluded that "There have been three epochs in the history of aphasia, each of which has been marked by a decided advance in knowledge."[44]

The first of these epochs was "*the Epoch of Broca*," which extended from 1864 to 1874. During this period "the claim of Broca that lesions of the posterior portion of the third frontal convolution on the left side produce a loss of speech was established upon an impregnable basis." In the second epoch—"*the epoch of Wernicke*, from 1874 to 1883"—the distinction between motor and sensory aphasia was recognized. This brought Starr to the third and current epoch in aphasia studies—*the epoch of* [Jean-Martin] *Charcot*—who, "with his sharp clinical insight and masterly power of analysis saw that further distinctions were possible."[45] Progress is here equated with the making of ever finer distinctions, a view of the point of aphasiological work that was quite typical (see chapter 3).

The last of Starr's epochs is more controversial than the other two: there would be some dispute as to whether Charcot's contribution was of such magnitude as to merit an eponymous era. However, the general features of his organization of aphasiological time are typical of what might be characterized as "textbook" history. Apart from an emphasis upon the crucial contributions made by outstanding individuals, the most salient feature of such history is its insistence on the cumulative, progressive nature of the growth of knowledge. Each giant stands on the shoulders of his predecessor in order to build an ever more imposing edifice.

Around 1900 some challenges to this optimistic, relatively uncomplicated narrative began to appear; aphasia studies reflected the widespread questioning of nineteenth-century certainties that occurred at the fin de siècle. Revisionist readings emerged in which the path to truth seemed more tortuous than had previously seemed the case; as well as heroes the story of aphasia studies, moreover, was now seen to have its villains who retarded rather than advanced knowledge. Truth might eventually win out but often it had first to triumph over much adversity.

Henry Head began his 1920 review of the aphasiological literature with an apparent endorsement of the metaphors of organic growth and the triumphalist tone that had dominated previous accounts. "The evolution of knowlege of cerebral localization," he declared, "is one of the most astonishing stories in the history of medicine."[46] Head went on to review

---

[44] M. Allen Starr, "Discussion of Cerebral Localization: Aphasia," *Transactions of the Congress of American Physicians and Surgeons* (New Haven: The Congress, 1889), p. 330.

[45] Ibid.

[46] Henry Head, "Aphasia: An Historical Review," *Brain* 43 (1920): 390–411, on p. 390.

the role of Gall, Bouillaud, and Broca in this story in a more or less conventional fashion. He then described the spread of interest in the question of aphasia to Britain, introducing a new character, John Hughlings Jackson, who debated the issue with Broca at the 1868 meeting of the British Association for the Advancement of Science. This early mention signalled Head's intention to repair the unfair neglect that Jackson's contributions to aphasiology had suffered in previous histories.

At this point Head's account began to diverge from the received version in more significant ways. Subsequent investigators, he charged, "took no care to emulate the clinical acumen of Broca or the psychological insight of Hughlings Jackson." Instead such aphasiologists as H. Charlton Bastian had proceeded along lines so ill-advised that they exerted an "evil influence on the subsequent course of the discussion." Bastian and his like were guilty of preferring facile procedures which led to error to the "difficulties and complexities" of Jackson's approach.[47]

The details of Head's attack on classical aphasiology are considered elsewhere in this book.[48] Here I wish only to point out how Head's work exemplifies a tendency in twentieth-century aphasia studies to use history as a polemical tool in the furtherance of various disciplinary programs. The controversy between so-called holist and localizationist neurologists has, in particular, involved tendentious readings of canonical aphasiological texts.

Thus in an 1960 paper Walther Riese also embraced Jackson as a prophet of sound aphasiological principles—although he observed that "Jackson himself did not grasp the full scope of his own observations."[49] Riese's aim was to illustrate the need for a more patient-centered, biographical approach to neurological disease especially when impairment of the higher, most distinctively human functions, was involved. Classic aphasiology's emphasis upon diagnosis rather than prognosis and therapy, and on anatomical localization rather than detailed patient history was a deviation from the proper concerns of clinical medicine. "Holist" neurologists, including Jackson, but more particularly continentals like Constantin von Monakow and Kurt Goldstein, had provided a necessary corrective to this unfortunate tendency.

Four years later Norman Geschwind described this version of events as "what to a very great extent has become the 'standard' history of aphasia." Geschwind called for a new revisionism. He had himself subscribed to this

[47] Ibid., p. 396.

[48] Head considerably expanded his history of the discipline in a later monograph: *Aphasia and Kindred Disorders of Speech*, 2 vols. (Cambridge: Cambridge University Press, 1926), vol. 1, pp. 1–141.

[49] Walther Riese, "Dynamics in Brain Lesions," in *Selected Papers on the History of Aphasia* (Amsterdam: Swets, 1977), pp. 70–85.

account but had come to see it as outrageously unfair to "people who had left their mark so indelibly in many areas of neurology." Geschwind found it impossible to believe that such figures as Wernicke, Bastian, and Charcot "could apparently have shown what was asserted to be the sheerest naivete and incompetence in the area of the higher functions."[50] It is noteworthy that whereas Riese was concerned at the historical neglect of the patient, Geschwind felt impelled to remedy injustices to the reputations of the great men of his profession.

Geschwind did not seek to denigrate the reputations of the neurologists on the "other," holistic side of the dichotomy posited by the standard history of aphasia. Goldstein too was a "great figure." What he did attempt was to minimize the differences between the localizationist and the holist schools—in effect to reinstate a version of the old view of the history of aphasia studies as a continuous process of gradual evolution.

One technique he adapted to this end was to subject one text— Goldstein's *Language and Language Disturbances*—to a close reading to show the inadequacy of the received notion of this author's work. This exercise revealed that if one ventured beyond the introductory theoretical section of the book to the more technical sections that followed, then it emerged that Goldstein was, in fact, "highly classical" in many of his statements on the representation of function in the cortex. Despite his avowed break with classical views on aphasia, Geschwind was able to quote passages which appeared to endorse views that "could have been written by the staunchest of classicists."[51] Such evident discrepancies raised the question, "Which is the real Kurt Goldstein?"[52]

Geschwind maintained that it *was* possible to discern the outlines of a "real" Goldstein lurking behind the cruces of the text. This assumption draws attention to some of the interpretative issues with which this book is concerned. Approaching a text in the expectation of finding an authorial essence is at best a highly problematic exercise. There will be much meaning in a text which is irreducible to any notion of authorial intent. That meaning is, moreover, never passively received but always actively constructed in acts of reading. The character, interests, and intentions of an author are always open to negotiation. The issue of these negotiations is identity.

The historiography of aphasia illustrates the divergent interpretations that this unfolding episode in the history of science and medicine has

---

[50] Norman Geschwind, "The Paradoxical Position of Kurt Goldstein in the History of Aphasia," in *Selected Papers on Language and the Brain* (Dordrecht: Reidel, 1974), pp. 62–72, on pp. 62–63.

[51] Ibid., pp. 67–68.

[52] Ibid., p. 69.

received. These various readings can be glossed in several ways. They can be seen as the expression of personal, disciplinary, regional, sectarian, or national interests; or as imbued with the notions of class and gender endemic in the cultures in which they were written. These readings also show how the history of aphasia has served as a space for the exposition of differing conceptions of the nature of medical science and of its relation to medical practice.

Humanistic notions that stress the need to preserve and respect the personality of a patient who has to some degree lost what is deemed a definitive human characteristic have conflicted with scientistic notions that seek to elide the individuality of any given case in the pursuit of universal natural laws. These competing ideals are not mutually exclusive; at certain moments in the dialectic they are, indeed, shown to be simply differences of emphasis or as different aspects of the same moral order.

In either case the moral order pertains to the profession charged with the study and management of those afflicted with aphasia. The speechless man or woman is fixed in a medical gaze whatever modulation of ethical rhetoric obtains at a given time or place. The persistent asymmetry in the power to produce narratives and representations is a more fundamental dichotomy in the literature of aphasia. It is, moreover, important to recognize this asymmetry as a *condition* of the science of aphasiology.[53] The corollary of the power exerted by the discourse over the voiceless patient is the empowerment of a community of practitioners made capable of generating a vast literature on the relations of language and the brain.[54]

My own readings of these texts have been informed by a number of interpretative resources. I depend heavily on Friedrich Nietzsche's notion of the inescapability of metaphor. My reliance on Michel Foucault's char-

[53] A perceptive rendition of this dichotomy is found in Pat Barker's novel *The Eye in the Door* (London: Penguin, 1994), p. 146: "[Rivers] watched Head's expression as he looked at Lucas's shaved scalp, and realized it differed hardly at all from his expression that morning as he'd bent over the cadaver. For the moment, Lucas had become simply a technical problem. Then Lucas looked up from his task, and instantly Head's face flashed open in his transforming smile. A murmur of encouragement, and Lucas returned to his drawing. Head's face, looking at the ridged purple scar on the shaved head, again became remote, withdrawn. His empathy, his strong sense of the humanity he shared with his patients, was again suspended. A necessary suspension, without which the practice of medical research, and indeed of medicine itself, would hardly be possible, but none the less identifiably the same suspension the soldier must achieve in order to kill."

[54] Corfield notes: "that language works through domination is open to challenge. Linguistic communication may equally encompass cooperation, convergence, and community." "Introduction," p. 24. Language can, however, function in *both* these modes depending on an individual's, or a category of individuals, situation within a discourse. See also Mario Biagioli's discussion of the role of discrete linguistic codes in the establishment of coherent and viable scientific communities: *Galileo, Courtier: The Practice of Science in the Culture of Absolutism* (Chicago: University of Chicago Press, 1993), pp. 241–44.

acterization of the power/knowledge nexus should also be apparent; it is indeed central to my account of the discourse of aphasia. I also owe a more general debt to such sociologically aware historians of science as Steven Shapin and Simon Schaffer. Their emphasis upon the rhetorical aspects of scientific writing and on the artifice involved in the demonstration of natural facts is reflected throughout this book. A rich body of literature in both art history and the sociology of science has guided my discussion of nonverbal representation in aphasia studies. Finally, *Lost Words* should be seen in the context of the recent tendency in the history of medicine, of which Roy Porter has been perhaps the foremost exponent, to seek to reinstate the patient's point of view—even if in the present instance this is chiefly a matter of articulating the ways in which the patient's point of view is *absent* from a body of medical literature.

Chapter 1 explores the emergence of the genre of the aphasiological case history. It contrasts two accounts of speech loss from the first half of the nineteenth century, both of which were written by medical men. The differences between the one that was to become canonical and the other that was relegated to a marginal status in the literature illustrate both what was definitive and what was systematically excluded from subsequent writing on aphasia.

While Lordat's and Bouillaud's "contributions" belong to the prehistory of aphasiology, chapter 2 deals with what is generally regarded as the originating moment of the enterprise proper: the 1861 debate at the Société d'Anthropologie at which Paul Broca first associated the faculty of articulate speech with the third frontal convolution of the brain. Through a study of this polyvocal text I seek to show some of the cultural ramifications of this discovery of the organic seat of language.

Chapter 3 treats the multiplicity of writing on aphasia in the period after 1861 as a single text with a collective authorship. These various contributions are seen as the surviving traces of the labour process that the discovery of a determinate relationship between language and the brain engendered. The chapter seeks in particular to identify the conditions that ensured the coherence and viability of this enterprise. As well as its literary aspects, the visual forms of representation employed in classical aphasiology are considered.

In contrast, chapters 4 and 5 deal with the writing on aphasia of two individuals, both of whom are usually regarded as somewhat at odds with the dominant tendency of aphasia studies. In the received history of the field John Hughlings Jackson figures as a neglected innovator whose efforts were unjustly neglected by contemporaries; their significance only became apparent in retrospect. What was said to distinguish Jackson's contribution to the field was his insistence on the need to consider the *psychological* aspects of aphasic disorders. Jackson attempted to give an account of the inner world of the aphasic: a narrative that was structured by assumptions about the dynamics of the mind fundamental to Western philosophy.

Henry Head's writings on aphasia make a natural complement to those of Jackson. It was largely due to Head's proselytizing that interest in Jackson's work was revived. Chapter 5 attempts to combine a more conventional approach to its protagonist with a close and critical reading of texts. Head saw his own contribution to aphasia studies as a continuation of Jackson's psychological approach to the subject. He maintained that the special circumstances surrounding his researches facilitated this endeavor. Head maintained that aphasias generated by wounds to the brain suffered by war casualties were especially instructive. Wounded *officers* were of particular heuristic value. Chapter 5 discusses the peculiar characteristics of the case histories that Head produced through his interactions with this class of patient. The chapter also considers the material and social technologies Head devised to produce serviceable three-dimensional representations of the inaccessible brains of these aphasics.

Chapter 6 also deals with writing that dissented from the orthodoxies of classic aphasiology. It analyzes well-known texts by Sigmund Freud and Pierre Marie that pay special attention to the use of metaphor, rhetorical strategies, and deployment of narrative devices with the aim of undermining some of the certainties of the discourse of aphasia. The account of Henri Bergson's discussion of aphasia reprises some of the themes of chapter 2; it shows how at the end of the nineteenth century the theme of language and the brain still possessed implications that transcended the domains of medicine and natural science narrowly conceived.

The seventh chapter deals with what amounts to a rather anomalous appendix to the aphasia literature. Reading the mass of these case histories one is struck by their emphasis upon diagnosis and classification; therapy scarcely merits a mention. By the 1880s, however, there was a burgeoning discussion of how the aphasic might through medical intervention be helped to recover at least part of his lost capacity. This discussion received a renewed impetus in the aftermath of the First World War when the medical profession, and society in general, was confronted with the problem of how to rehabilitate large numbers of soldiers who had suffered head wounds. The most dramatic remedy was direct surgical intervention. However, treatment usually took the form of speech therapy which often extended over considerable periods of time. Texts describing these regimes provide a view of both patient and practitioner that differs in important respects from that inscribed in the main body of the aphasia canon. By means of ingenious techniques the aphasic is made to utter new truths about his condition; but at the same time the doctor reveals previously unknown sides to his nature.

ONE

CONSTRUING SILENCE

The exact sciences constitute a monologic form of knowledge:
the intellect contemplates a *thing* and expounds upon it.
There is only one subject here—cognizing (contemplating)
and speaking (expounding). In opposition to the subject
there is only a *voiceless thing*.
(Mikhail Bakhtin, Speech Genres and
Other Late Essays, *p. 161.)*

IN THE SUMMER of 1825 Jacques Lordat (1773–1870), a medical
practitioner and professor of anatomy and physiology at Montpellier,
suffered a prolonged bout of illness. By the fifteenth day most of the
symptoms, apart from a slight fever and a "heaviness" of the head, had
disappeared. But then a new and alarming development occurred: "I became conscious that when I wished to speak I did not find the expressions
that I required." This "symptom surprised me and made me thoughtful";
Lordat sought comfort in the hope that this was merely a transient state
of affairs.

While preoccupied with these reflections, he was informed of the arrival
of a visitor to inquire after his health:

> I opened my mouth to reply to this courtesy. The thought was quite ready,
> but the sounds which should have confided it to the intermediary were no
> longer at my disposal. I turned round in consternation, and I said, to myself
> [*en moi-même*]: *So it is true that I can no longer speak!*[1]

A few months earlier Jean-Baptiste Bouillaud (1796–1881), a Paris physician, had read a paper to the Académie Royale de Médecine in which he
argued that loss of speech was invariably associated with a lesion of the
frontal lobes of the brain. He adduced several cases drawn both from his
own clinical experience and from that of others to support his claim to

---

[1] Jacques Lordat, "Analyse de la parole pour servir à la théorie de divers cas d'ALALIE et
de PARALALIE (de mutisme et d'imperfection du parler) que les nosologistes ont mal
connu," *Journal de la Société de Médecine-Pratique de Montpellier* 7 (1843): 333–353; 417–
433, p. 347.

have located the "legislative organ of speech."[2] Bouillaud was to repeat and elaborate this thesis in a number of subsequent publications.[3]

Both these episodes may be viewed as early chapters in the nineteenth-century medical discourse about language. Lordat was quite explicit that his intent was not merely to record the facts of his own case, but also to lay a theoretical foundation upon which a medical understanding of the human faculty of language could be built. The origins of language were beyond the legitimate bounds of medicine; it was, however, perfectly proper for medicine to ask how human beings made use of the languages they possessed. Nor was this a purely speculative line of inquiry: a detailed analysis of the mechanisms of language was required so that "the theory of speech is of use in the practice of medicine." To whom, he asked rhetorically, could those afflicted with some speech defect turn "if not to the doctor when it is a question of determining the form of the affliction, the nature of its cause, [and] the designation of the remedy if one exists?"[4]

From a twentieth-century perspective, however, Lordat's attempt to enhance the medical understanding of language appear anomalous and strangely deficient. In the words of a modern editor, "what is, without doubt, most astonishing about Lordat's [paper] is the absence of anatomo-clinical references."[5] While Lordat's text merits inclusion alongside Bouillaud's address in a collection on "The Birth of the Neuropsychology of Language," it is reproduced merely as a curiosity. Its principal interest resides in the accident that Lordat was both a medical practitioner and someone with personal experience of language loss.

Bouillaud's "Recherches Cliniques" possesses an altogether different status. It is a classic text within the historiography of aphasia studies. Bouillaud's methods and conclusions might be in some respects defective

---

[2] Jean-Baptiste Bouillaud, "Recherches cliniques propres à démontrer que la perte de la parole correspond à la lésion des lobules antérieurs du cerveau, et à confirmer l'opinion de M. GALL, sur le siège de l'organe du langage articulé," *Archives Générales de Médecine* 8 (1825): 25–45, p. 30.

[3] Jean-Baptiste Bouillaud, *Traité clinique et physiologique de l'encéphalite, ou inflammation du cerveau, et de ses suites, telles que le ramollissement, la suppuration, les abcès, les tubercules, le squirrhe, le cancer, etc.* (Paris: J.-B. Baillière, 1825); idem, "Exposition de nouveaux faits à l'appui de l'opinion qui localise dans les lobules antérieures du cerveau le principe législateur de la parole; examen préliminaire des objections dont cette opinion a été le sujet," *Bullétin de l'Académie Royale de Médecine* 4 (1839–40): 282–328; idem, "Recherches cliniques propres à démontrer que le sens du langage articulé et le principe coordinateur des mouvements de la parole résident dans les lobules antérieurs du cerveau," *Bull. Acad. Roy. de Méd.* 1er trimestre (1848): 699–719.

[4] Lordat, "Analyse," pp. 333–335.

[5] H. Hecaen and J. Dubois, *La naissance de la neuropsychologie du langage 1825–1865* (Paris: Flammarion, 1969), p. 168.

(because, for instance, of his failure to recognize the phenomenon of lateralization[6]); but his endeavor is nonetheless accorded a seal of authenticity denied Lordat's efforts. Bouillaud is thus credited with having "laid the foundation for the classification of aphasia as it was to be developed later by Broca, Wernicke, and Lichtheim."[7] Samuel Greenblatt expressed this foundational status more tersely when he identified Bouillaud's writing as the primal *Logos* of aphasia studies: "in the beginning there was Bouillaud."[8]

Such accolades tend to stress the clinical foundations of Bouillaud's theories on the physiopathology of language. His status as a practicing physician distinguishes him from such merely "speculative thinkers" as Franz Josef Gall. But Lordat was also a clinician. A lack of experience does not explain his exclusion from the canon, but rather the *kind* of experience that he distilled from his encounters with patients—including the occasion when he was his own patient.

The basic experiential unit from which both Bouillaud and Lordat obtained the justification for their respective views on the nature of language was the case history. In other words, they both relied upon narratives of particular episodes of illness to demonstrate or instance more general truths. But the notion of a shared "clinical" basis to their endeavors is misleading because it fails to take into account the discrepancy between the narrative forms that appear in their respective texts.

The centrality of narrative in the composition of medical knowledge is a point that no longer needs to be labored.[9] What should, however, be emphasized is that narrative does not present a single way of knowing the patient or the disease. There are on the contrary a multiplicity of narrative forms in which very different patients and diseases can be constituted as legitimate objects of knowledge. The "clinical reality" to which rhetorical appeal is so regularly made is therefore an historically contingent entity.

The nature of that reality depends upon the mode of representation embodied in any particular form of case history. Insofar as stable forms of representational convention exist in any given context it is possible to speak of *genres* of case history. An examination of the case histories de-

---

[6] See, for example: Anne Harrington, *Medicine, Mind, and the Double Brain: A Study in Nineteenth-Century Thought* (Princeton: Princeton Univ. Press, 1987), pp. 54–55.

[7] Otto M. Marx, "Aphasia Studies and Language Theory in the 19th Century," *Bulletin of the History of Medicine* 40 (1966): 328–349, p. 337.

[8] Samuel H. Greenblatt, "Hughlings Jackson's First Encounter with the Work of Paul Broca: The Physiological and Philosophical Background," *Bulletin of the History of Medicine* 44 (1970): 555–570, on p. 569.

[9] See: Kathryn Montgomery Hunter, *Doctors' Stories: The Narrative Structure of Medical Knowledge* (Princeton: Princeton Univ. Press, 1991).

ployed by Lordat and by Bouillaud reveal differences so profound as to justify their classification into distinct genres. A literary genre may be considered as both an enabling and as an inhibitory device: it facilitates certain discursive possibilities while precluding or at least hindering others. Genres perform a regulatory role with respect to individual utterance: "they have a normative significance for the the speaking individuum, and they are not created by him but are given to him."[10] The use of language within a genre is therefore as much a performative as merely a descriptive act; it creates the reality that it describes. An ability to write *within* a particular genre may, moreover, be a qualification for participation in a given way of life.

Bouillaud's cases are exemplary of a literary tradition that was to become dominant, indeed exclusive, within modern Western medicine. More specifically, they supply a prototype for the case histories upon which later nineteenth- and twentieth-century aphasiology depended. A mark of the success of this tradition is that the representational artifice that these histories embody has become entirely transparent; they seem to provide an altogether natural and inevitable account of the clinical world. Their status as a literary genre has been effectively suppressed.

In contrast Lordat's cases appear quaint or deviant to the modern eye; they are, as we have seen, in any event deemed to be in crucial respects defective. The following section seeks to characterize the distinctive representational conventions that define Lordat's accounts of diseased speech. A contrast with the conventions at work in Bouillaud's narratives should then serve to emphasize their partial and artifactual nature. The silences of the canonical neurological case history will be seen to be as significant as what it allows to be said.

Talking to Your Self; Talking to Other Selves

Lordat described the circumstances of his case in a course of lectures on physiology that he gave at Montpellier in the 1842–43 session. He prefaced his account with a theoretical statement of the acts necessary for thought to be transmuted into the sounds that are its vehicle. Lordat distinguished no less than ten such preliminary steps; such a minute analysis was justified by the clinical importance of the subject. Every day, he declared,

---

[10] M. M. Bakhtin, "The Problem of Speech Genres," in *Speech Genres and Other Late Essays*, trans. Vern W. McGee, (Austin: University of Texas Press, 1986), pp. 60–102, on pp. 80–81.

we are consulted about defects in the exercise of language. Defects of this function humiliate those who suffer from them; sometimes they suffice to impede the unions that give life its charm; they render one incompetent for the diverse professions for which one had been destined by society, by nature, and by birth.[11]

In short, this affliction prevented an individual from exercising personality.

Lordat saw the healthy exercise of language as dependent upon the cooperation and persistence of a due relation between the three elements of a person: the intellect or *sens intime*, the vital force, and the body. Speech represented a "corporification" of ideas. It was a "truly admirable mental operation to clad modes of the intellect in bodies capable of transmission among living persons or for perpetuity!—That is what we do continually when we speak or write."[12] Speech was thus an act by which the mind showed its power over the material.

What, however, would be the situation of a person whose *sens intime* remained unaltered, but in whom the vital force lost the faculty of finding the sounds in which to dress his or her thoughts? Such an individual would continue to think as before; he could still arrange and analyze his ideas. When, however,

> he requires from the vital force the memory of the sounds that serve as signs, it cannot provide him with any. He is impotent in speech: despite a sound consciousness, a normal intellect, and healthy vocal organs, he is afflicted with *alalia*, with an impossibility of speaking.[13]

Nor was this merely a speculative possibility. There were numerous instances of such dumbness—"among which I have had the misfortune and have today the advantage to be counted."[14] From a general discussion of the dynamics of language Lordat thus proceeded to his own case. The disjunction was not, however, absolute. Lordat's theory of speech, although highly general, was also personal inasmuch as it supplied a model by means of which the individual consciousness could comprehend what passed within it. He had accordingly employed this system to elucidate what had occurred within him in the course of his attack of "alalia."

But Lordat's narrative did not commence with this episode itself. Instead he began by remarking that he had since the age of ten been subject to periodic attacks of quinsey which occasioned excessive salivation and culminated in tonsilar suppuration. Up to the age of twenty-one this affliction had occurred every two or three years; thereafter, it was an annual

---

[11] Lordat, "Analyse," p. 334.
[12] Ibid., p. 341.
[13] Ibid., pp. 344–345.
[14] Ibid., p. 343.

event always appearing in the same months. As he aged the attacks became less frequent, but still sometimes occurred during the summer.[15]

This prolegomenon on Lordat's medical history is followed by an account of the events of the summer of 1825. On 17 July, after long mental exertion and anxiety, he suffered his usual quinsey. The disease then took a different turn: restlessness, insomnia, and a slight fever supervened upon the original symptoms. After the third day Lordat found it impossible to swallow. This state of affairs lasted a week after which Lordat *seemed* to be cured. But, in his capacity as a medical practitioner rather than sufferer, he received the congratulations of his friends on his recovery with some skepticism. He knew that he had experienced a delitescence rather than a genuine cure. These suspicions were confirmed when two days later he was afflicted by severe abdominal pains.[16]

After a further week these symptoms were in turn replaced by a fever and "heaviness" of the head. It was then that Lordat first noticed difficulties with his speech. Within twenty-four hours this had grown to the point that: "I found myself bereft of the value of almost all words. If a few remained to me, they were virtually useless to me because I no longer remembered the manner of coordination necessary for the expression of a thought." He was no more capable of comprehending the significance of the sounds he heard others express.[17]

Lordat's narrative thus took the form of a number of interlocking temporal sequences: first the history of his health over the duration of his life; then the course of the illness he suffered in the summer of 1825; and lastly the story of the alalia itself. The more particular is to be read in the context of the more general narrative; taken together they provide a unified and coherent story. By embedding the alalia within this framework Lordat stipulated the terms in which it was to be understood; the illness was to be seen not as an isolated event but as part of the history of an individual who had unity and persistency through time. This entity was a self that Lordat was able to recognize as his.[18]

The emphasis upon periodic attacks of quinsey in the course of his life, for example, casts a particular light upon Lordat's later illness. It establishes a propensity of the embodied self for disease of the organs most immediately involved in speech of which the alalia might be considered as

---

[15] Ibid., pp. 345–346.

[16] Ibid., p. 346.

[17] Ibid., p. 347.

[18] On the role of temporal succession in the constitution of the modern self see: Huck Gutman, "Rousseau's *Confessions*: A Technology of the Self," in Luther H. Martin, Huck Gutman, Patrick H. Hutton (eds.), *Technologies of the Self: A Seminar with Michel Foucault* (Amherst: University of Massachussetts Press, 1988), pp. 99–120, pp. 100–101.

a special manifestation. In one passage Lordat writes of the self [*moi*] as the setting within which the pathological events he describes occur.[19]

This self was, moreover, an affective object as well as a heuristic device. The concept embodied Lordat's sense of identity and personal worth; from this perspective, the lesion it had now suffered was especially afflicting. Lordat asked his audience to imagine

> the position of a man who, from his station in life, is in continuous relation with others by means of speech, and who, while retaining all his usual mental aptitudes and intellectual needs, finds himself sequestered from his fellows by consciousness [*par le sens intime*] even though he lives in their midst. He is witness to their mutual relations, he feel himself equal to them, and [yet] a cruel fate prevents him from entering into their intercourse.[20]

Nor could he take any comfort in the written word: "in losing the memory of heard words, I had lost that of visual signs. . . . I do not tell you of my despair, you should surmise it."[21] The capacity for language was thus a critical aspect of Lordat's concept of self; its loss was a serious, almost deadly, blow to the integrity of that concept.

As distressing as was his own apperception of infirmity, the imagination of how others would now view his self is presented as yet more painful. Lordat was preoccupied with a sentiment of the incongruity between what he truly was, as a *sens intime*, and of how he must in his altered state appear to others. He felt that the difficulty of taking part in the conversations that he witnessed must "give to my visage an expression of sombre stupor which sometimes inspired a vain and insulting pity." He tried to recuperate some self-respect with the thought that his inferiority was more apparent than real; to retain this comforting idea, however, he needed to believe that his present condition was only temporary.[22]

After some weeks of "profound sadness and resignation," Lordat noticed a change in his condition. On regarding from a distance the spine of one of the books in his library, "I noticed . . . that I read clearly the title *Hippocratis Opera*. This discovery made me shed tears of joy."[23] He then set about the task of relearning speech and writing. Lordat had returned to his former self. The fact that the book which occasioned the beginnings of Lordat's recovery was not only a medical work but, in the Western tradition, *the* foundational medical text is also worthy of remark. Renewed access to such works marked the return of the crucial professional dimension of Lordat's identity.

---

[19] Lordat, "Analyse," p. 345.
[20] Ibid., p. 348.
[21] Ibid., p. 351.
[22] Ibid., p. 350.
[23] Ibid., p. 351.

This self had, however, undergone a permanent transformation as a result of the degradation it had experienced. Lordat intermingled his grammatical reeducation with a study of cases similar to the illness he had just suffered. He realized that "doctors have badly understood and described them: it is necessary to have been a sufferer in order to make a true diagnosis."[24] His own experience of alalia gave him, in short, a special competence as a medical practitioner when confronted with similar complaints in others. This claim that a direct phenomenological experience of the affliction was a condition for its proper understanding is among the most salient ways in which Lordat's approach differed from what was to become the dominant mode of explicating language loss. Lordat proceeded to recount a number of subsequent instances in his practice to substantiate this claim.

What is noteworthy about these histories is that in them Lordat treats these others as other *selves*: he accords them the same status that he did to the simultaneous observer and subject of his own illness. When dealing with other sufferers Lordat assumed the same epistemological stance by which he had divined the nature of his own case; he learned by a dialogue with the self in question. Given the fact that some of his patients were entirely dumb, this dialogic strategy confronted severe practical difficulties; but there were other means of determining the character of a self and of its disease than by direct conversation. Two examples will suffice to give the character of these case histories.

The first of these is the case of "The late M. MOULINIER, [a] most distinguished landscape painter, . . . [who] was struck two or three years before his death, by a sudden and simple verbal amnesia which lasted no more than some twenty-six hours." Most of the narrative is recounted from the patient's perspective. Moulinier had gone to stay with a friend in the country in order to paint a landscape. He

> took a light lunch of bread and an orange, and made his way to the designated place. He promptly set to work. He was in the open air, under the sun, furnished with a large hat. While sketching he had need to give an order to a servant who was nearby; he realized that he had forgotten the name of this individual, he cried out, and when he wished to express the order, he saw that he had not a word at his command. This discovery astonished and terrified him.[25]

He experienced no other symptoms.

Troubled, Moulinier returned home wishing to be with his family. Lordat was called to attend him; it is at this stage only that the doctor appears in the story. At this point the perspective ceases to be that of the patient

---

[24] Ibid., pp. 351–352.
[25] Ibid., p. 422.

and becomes that of his medical attendant. But it is important to stress that the doctor's view remains a distinct element within the narrative; it supplements rather than subsumes other voices within it. Lordat marks his entry into the case quite clearly:

> I was called. I find him in bed, surprised, impatient, vexed. He cannot say a word. I question him: he lets me know that he is perfectly healthy—apart from this symptom. I explain to him the nature of his muteness; he responds by means of signs that it is just so.[26]

After consultation with other practitioners it is decided to bleed the patient—not because this remedy is thought to be of any use, but "only out of human respect."[27]

Lordat visited Moulinier on the following day and found that his voice had returned. Moulinier "was able to tell all that had happened to him and all the thoughts [*idées*] that he had had." The narrative thus ends with a dialogue between patient and doctor in which the latter explicitly acknowledges that the former is the prime source of what has gone before. In particular, the patient's consciousness—his *sens intime*—is recognized as an important repository of narrative detail.

The second example concerns a priest, wrongly diagnosed as having suffered an apoplectic attack, who was in fact afflicted with a *paraamnésie* for words. As in the other case the narrative is prefaced with information about the *curé's* circumstances and station which help to establish him as a social actor prior and ulterior to his condition as a patient. Again, Lordat's first appearance is well-marked:

> When I arrived the supposed apoplectic was seated on his bed wide awake; he received me with a courteous and open manner. He seemed more concerned about me than about himself. I had come on horseback; the weather was bad. He made signs to indicate that I should first get warm and have a meal. This language, silent as it was, was sufficiently significant that everyone moved and obeyed.[28]

Lordat is therefore received in the first instance not merely as a doctor but as a guest; his patient is also his host. This serves to give depth and complexity to the relationship between the two; but it serves also reinforce the *curé's* status as a self whose existence is not exhausted by his status as a patient. Unlike Moulinier he could, for instance, still give orders to his servants—an important aspect of his social identity—although, as the later narrative makes clear, not without difficulty.

[26] Ibid.
[27] Ibid., pp. 422–423.
[28] Ibid., pp. 425–426.

The point is reinforced by the remainder of the account. The *curé* attempted to give a further order which no one could understand: "He showed his impatience by two very vigorous words, of which one was *i*, and the other the most forceful swearword in our language, which begins with an *f*." These cries were repeated until the *curé's* meaning was at last divined by those present. Lordat subsequently discovered that his patient always expressed his frustration by the use of these interjections; but this was evidence of the pathological state of his speech: "As he was a man of spirit and a priest, I thought that he was ignorant of the meaning of the terms that he pronounced."[29] In short, the *curé's* illness had caused the same kind of discrepancy between the authentic self and the manifest self that occurred in Lordat's own case; his body had failed him.

Lordat in fact came across this patient before his own alalia, and at the time he did not fully appreciate the significance of the symptoms that he encountered. When, however, he was himself taken ill Lordat asked the *curé* to visit him in the hope of learning more of the nature of the condition with which both were afflicted. The physician thus acknowledged a symmetry between himself and his former patient. Lordat found that although the priest was still deprived of the use of French, he could now converse in his local patois; but he remained unable to read since his accident and had conversed only with his servants and with peasants.[30]

Lordat's alalia was therefore a disease that struck well-defined selves, who possessed a life history, a social station, and established capacities. These characteristics are established by the inclusion of detail about these individuals redundant to their status as mere patients. They are allowed their own voice in the case history; even when Lordat appears, his perspective does not dominate to the exclusion of others. A genuine dialogic pluralism is preserved.

From a modern viewpoint these narratives are at once perplexing and infuriating. On the one hand, they seem to offer a wealth of superfluous detail: why, for instance, should we be told what Moulinier had for lunch on the day of his attack? On the other hand, they are frustratingly silent on matters which *should* appear in a clinical history; we are left to guess as to why the *curé's* condition was wrongly thought to be of an apoplectic nature. There is a pervasive lack of interest in recording physical signs.

Lordat was dismissive of attempts to supply a anatomico-pathological dimension to his narratives: "For a long time one has only spoken of fluxions, of congestions, of irritations, of inflammations, of swellings, of alterations in the substance of parts: I found nothing of the sort in my ill-

---

[29] Ibid., p. 426.
[30] Ibid., pp. 426–427.

ness."[31] He conceded that in many cases of the "amnesia" with which he was concerned, evidence of organic change in the brain was visible after death; but he regarded this as a concomitant or complication rather than as a cause of the symptoms with which he was most concerned.[32] By minimizing the need to correlate symptoms with postmortem appearances, Lordat placed himself at odds with the central tenets of "Paris Medicine," a system that was constitutive of the nineteenth-century clinic.[33]

An analogy with pictorial representation is instructive in trying to define the distinctive aspect of these case histories and in establishing how they differ from those that follow. To adapt terms used by Svetlana Alpers in her study of seventeenth-century Dutch painting, Lordat's narratives are marked by an absence of a "prior frame"—at least, that border is distinctly fuzzy. They are also characterized by "the frequent absence of a positioned viewer"; the perspective shifts in the course of the history. Redundant details such as Moulinier's orange also testify to a impulse to describe "the world seen," rather than to shape an account to some predetermined end.[34] When we come to consider Bouillaud's case histories we will see an inversion of these biases.

Lordat's Philosophy of Medicine

By going beyond the single text by Lordat so far considered it is possible to render the biases and silences evident in his clinical histories somewhat more intelligible. In various writings arising from his pedagogical activities in Montpellier he attempted to elaborate a distinctive concept of medical epistemology. This was a decidedly polemical endeavor: Lordat's aim was not only to set forth his own notions of the foundations of medical knowledge and practice, but also to discredit what he saw as a rival and pernicious system.[35]

---

[31] Ibid., p. 352.

[32] Ibid., p. 421.

[33] On Paris Medicine see: Erwin H. Ackerknecht, *Medicine at the Paris Hospital* (Baltimore: Johns Hopkins University, 1967); Russell C. Maulitz, *Morbid Appearances: The Anatomy of Pathology in the Early Nineteenth Century* (Cambridge: Cambridge University Press, 1987); Caroline Hannaway and Ann La Berge, *Rethinking Paris Medicine* (Amsterdam: Rodopi, 1999).

[34] Svetlana Alpers, *The Art of Describing: Dutch Art in the Seventeenth Century* (London: Penguin Books, 1989), p. xxv. Lordat wrote on the visual arts and their relevance to medical education.

[35] On Lordat's attempt to assert the claims of the Montpellier tradition against the hegemonic pretensions of Parisian medical culture see: Elizabeth A. Williams, *The Physical and the Moral: Anthropology, Physiology, and Philosophical Medicine in France, 1750–1850* (Cambridge: Cambridge University Press, 1994), pp. 136–140.

He told his students that everything he said about his own doctrine was to be viewed "in parallel with that of the Doctors who style themselves *Organicists*, that is with the opinion of those who claim to find in the anatomy of organs sufficient reason for all that takes place in man. . . . This Organicist School is the enemy of ours."[36] He did not imagine that he could convert the adherents of this hostile school with his arguments; the difference between them was too absolute for any reconciliation. His enemies, Lordat claimed, themselves suffered from a kind of word blindness: "they do not even grammatically understand either our propositions or their connexions."[37]

Lordat presented himself as the defender of a medical tradition that had long had its seat in Montpellier; its most notable proponent had been Paul-Joseph Barthez.[38] At the core of this doctrine was a recognition of the need to acknowledge the plurality of human nature. Man was not merely a body; his organism was a compound of spiritual, vital, and material components—"hence the inadequacy of Anatomy." Consequently, it behooved medicine to adopt a form of epistemological pluralism: "We seek *all* the causes, and we study the invisible with as much zeal and conscientiousness as we study the visible"; the organicists, in contrast, "wish only to occupy themselves with the material, and have a horror of the invisible." Certain truths were not, however, present to the clinical gaze. Medical practice must also be informed by a recognition of the complexity of its subject; it was necessary to appreciate the true needs of the concrete patient rather than to be content with tending to those of an abstraction.[39]

Lordat characterized his opponents as "Cartesians" because they recognized only two substances in the universe and ignored the existence of a peculiar vital realm. In fact, even this dualism tended to collapse in the face of the organicists' insistence on simplification; consciousness itself could be referred to an "arrangement of matter."[40] In their obsession with anatomy, the organicists mistook conditions for causes; and they "violated the rules of Natural Philosophy by refusing to distinguish between different kinds of causality."[41]

---

[36] Jacques Lordat, *Essai d'une caractéristique de l'enseignement médicale de Montpellier, développée dans les quatre premières leçons du cours de physiologie de l'année scolaire 1841–1842* (Paris: J.-B. Baillière, 1843), p. 6.

[37] Ibid., p. 10.

[38] On Barthez' vitalism see: François Duchesneau, "Vitalism in Late Eighteenth-Century Physiology: The Cases of Barthez, Blumenbach and John Hunter," in W. F. Bynum and Roy Porter (eds.), *William Hunter and the Eighteenth-Century Medical World* (Cambridge: Cambridge University Press, 1985), pp. 260–269.

[39] Lordat, *Essai d'une caractéristique*, p. 11.

[40] Ibid., pp. 23–24.

[41] Ibid., p. 33.

The inadequacies of the organicists were perhaps most apparent in the defective forms of narrative that proceeded from their premises. Lordat compared them to a

> geographer who, on the occasion of a political revolution or of a great battle of which he wishes to know the moral causes, diverts us from this research by occupying us with the locations where this took place, with the physical circumstances and material effects which co-existed with the events.[42]

The geographical metaphor to which Lordat alluded was to loom large in the nineteenth-century exploration of the brain (see chapter 3).

Lordat's principal objection was, therefore, to the monistic, reductionist aspect of his enemies' system. Not only their concept of the living body, but also their notion of the nature of medical knowledge, which sought to impose on medicine a single natural scientific way of knowing, was flawed. Lordat did not deny that an anatomical understanding of the body was of use in medicine; to rely solely upon knowledge derived in this fashion was, however, to neglect other no less important aspects of the medical subject.

He urged the necessity of an *aesthetic* as well as a scientific aspect to medical understanding. The study of painting was, he maintained, a valuable adjunct to a medical education because it developed in the physician a sensitivity to the immaterial but nonetheless real aspects of human nature with which he would have to deal in practice. For this reason, "when one seeks to discover in a pictorial representation the modes of feeling [*modes pathétiques*] the artist wanted to express, one makes better use of one's time, and one is nearer to the . . . science of man, considered as a living and thinking [being], that when one seeks to reduce willy-nilly vital phenomena to mechanical laws."[43]

In his "Analyse de Parole" Lordat made no reference to Bouillaud's extensively discussed publications on the subject. Bouillaud does, however, often figure in other of Lordat's writings as a representative of the organicist school—and, more specifically, of a particularly virulent strain of this movement associated with the doctrines of François-Joseph-Victor Broussais.[44] Lordat objected not only to the content of this doctrine but to the language with which its supporters chose to articulate their claims.[45]

[42] Ibid., p. 34.

[43] Jacques Lordat, *Essai sur l'iconologie médicale, ou sur les rapports d'utilité qui existent entre l'art du dessin et l'étude de la médecine* (Montpellier: Picot, 1833), p. 48.

[44] The best account of Broussais and his school is found in: Jean-François Braunstein, *Broussais et le matérialisme: médecine et philosophie au XIXe siècle* (Paris: Méridiens Klinck-sieck, 1986).

[45] Jacques Lordat, *Leçons de physiologie, extraites du cours fait à la faculté de Médecine de Montpellier, dans le semèstre de 1835 à 1836* (Paris: Baillière, 1837), pp. 13–14.

Bouillaud had in the course of an introductory lecture of 1835 spoken of a *revolution* set in train by Broussais which had completely overthrown the existing medical edifice. Lordat took exception to Bouillaud's choice of so culturally loaded a word. He also objected to Bouillaud's use of military metaphors in this discourse; Lordat promised his students that no such ferocious rhetoric would be found in *his* teaching—"because I do not wish to deploy you in battle nor to lead you to Thermopylae."[46] The use of such language in an academic setting was abhorrent because it smacked of a polemic appropriate not to reasoning individuals but "to the masses."[47]

These remarks give some insight into the wider cultural connotations of Lordat's repudiation of organicism.[48] He saw this system as tainted by a revolutionary ideology—as a manifestation of a kind of medical Jacobinism—which called for fundamental change and which glorified conflict. The former fault was especially obnoxious to a conservative sensibility: Lordat reproached

> the medical reformers for having interrupted the succession between the past and the present, and of having wished to form a new science which had nothing in common with what has gone before. . . . In true progress there are no leaps. The present ought to be the continuation of the past, just as the future will be the continuation of the present.[49]

There are obvious affinities between Lordat's own ideas—particularly his concept of the living body—and aspects of early nineteenth-century conservative thought. He had eschewed the use of terms such as "organic," "organization," and "organism," because of the abuse they had suffered. Organization, properly understood, signified no more than an instrument of the agents that employed it.[50] Lordat's own concept of man as a compound of three elements—mind, vital force, and matter—conformed to the Bonaldian triad of Power—Instrument—Servant.[51]

---

[46] Ibid., pp. 15, 27. A battle, of course, in which the Spartan army was slaughtered.

[47] Ibid., p. 276. A similar disdain for the *foule* was to appear in the writings of Pierre Marie in the early twentieth century: see chapter 6.

[48] I have considered the relations between medical and political philosophy in post-revolutionary France more fully in: "Medical Science and Moral Science: The Cultural Relations of Physiology in Restoration France," *History of Science* 25 (1987): 111–46.

[49] Lordat, *Leçons*, pp. 284–285.

[50] Jacques Lordat, *Ébauche du plan d'un traité complète de physiologie humaine, adressée à M. Caizergues, doyen de la Faculté de Médecine de Montpellier* (Montpellier: Castel, 1841), pp. 10–11.

[51] Lordat later acknowledged this affinity with Bonald's thought: Jacques Lordat, *Idée pittoresque de la physiologie humain médicale enseignée à Montpellier* (Montpellier: Ricard Frères, 1849), pp. 16–17. For an outline of Bonaldian philosophy see: W. Jay Reedy, "Lan-

Lordat himself drew out this analogy by characterizing the constituent elements of human nature as: "Consciousness [*sens intime*], Sovereign; Vital Force, Executant; Material Aggregate, Instrument."[52] He went to some lengths to establish the legitimacy of transferring terms and concepts from one realm, such as the social, to another, the vital.[53] In the case of speech the sovereign mind employed the vocal organs to express its thoughts; alalia was therefore a form of rebellion by the organs over their lawful master.[54]

Lordat's medical philosophy can thus be seen as one expression of a nineteenth-century conservative revulsion against the French Revolution and its far-ranging cultural consequences. His critique of the partial vision of disease, of the patient, and of the physician's role embodied in "organicism" was, moreover, to be repeated throughout the nineteenth century and beyond in attacks upon the model that had come to dominate Western medicine.

Lordat located Bouillaud and the organicist school of which he was a representative within the modernist tendency that he so deplored. He implied that the clinical consciousness of the organicist was flawed because of his faulty understanding of the human body and fallacious notions of medical epistemology. Lordat did not, however, seek to substantiate these claims by an investigation of the site where the effect of such obductions and partialities of clinical vision might be most apparent: in the case histories composed by his enemies.

Medicine as Science

Lordat's characterization of organicism inevitably contained elements of caricature; his aim was to underline what he saw as the most egregious aspects of the system. He nonetheless isolated certain concepts and rhetorical stances key to the school's thinking. Bouillaud did espouse a saltatory theory of scientific progress: knowledge advanced by "great and fortunate scientific revolutions," not by the gradual adaptation and improvement of a prior body of learning. Moreover, he saw heroic, Napoleonic figures—of whom Broussais was the outstanding example—as crucial to these benign upheavals in science.[55]

---

guage, Counter-Revolution and the 'Two Cultures': Bonald's Traditionalist Scientism," *Journal of the History of Ideas* 44 (1983): 579–97.

[52] Lordat, *Ébauche*, p. 114.

[53] Ibid., p. 49.

[54] It is in this context worth drawing attention to the master/servant motif that figures in Lordat's case histories.

[55] Bouillaud, *Traité*, pp. v–vi.

Different sciences achieved their climactic revolution at different epochs; a certain maturity was necessary before the final stage in the intellectual ascent of a discipline could be reached. While physics and chemistry had forged ahead, Bouillaud complained that medicine had for too long remained "immobile in the midst of the general movement of improvement which swept along the other sciences." This period of stagnation was, however, at last coming to an end: medicine too was on the march.[56]

Bouillaud thus adopted a positivist model of medical progress. He privileged a particular way of knowing—that most perfectly exemplified in the physical sciences—and maintained that medicine would advance in proportion to its assimilation of this method. Bouillaud looked forward to the "the happy time when medicine will, like chemistry, possess a fixed and uniform language!" He quoted Condillac's dictum that sciences were in essence "well-made languages."[57] Lordat would, no doubt, have seen in this insistence on a "fixed and uniform" medical language a further symptom of the modernist delusion to which organicism was subject; the map of medical knowledge that had been gradually established over centuries was to be suddenly redrawn on new first principles.

Bouillaud's prediction of an imminent unified language of medical discourse possessed a visionary, rhetorical quality. A degree of uniformity in the linguistic practices of clinical medicine was, however, evident by the 1820s. The stability of these usages had not been imposed upon medicine from above by some enlightened despot, but had emerged through a more subtle and elusive process. This linguistic regime nonetheless exerted power over all those involved in the work of the clinic. A scientistic conception of medicine had become inscribed upon the documentary practices of the clinic—upon the way the "case" itself was composed.

On scientistic premises medicine was, above all, an enterprise of discovery: the clinician's primary concern was with the delivery of new "contributions" to the fund of knowledge. Clinical medicine was thus merely an adjunct of physiology. In Bouillaud's words,

> You can now see how the study of diseases can serve to uncover the most profound physiological mysteries. In effect, diseases may be considered as experiments, as kinds of *vivisections*, performed upon man by nature herself.[58]

The notion of disease as natural experiment was to become a common trope in the nineteenth century; the analogy had the effect of approximat-

[56] Ibid., p. vi.
[57] Ibid., p. xii.
[58] Ibid., pp. xxi–xxii.

ing the clinic to the laboratory and of identifying the role of physician
with that of the scientist. The patient in turn was tacitly assigned the status
of an experimental subject.

On this model, the analytic, diagnostic aspect of clinical practice was
paramount; it led to universal truths that transcended any individual case.
Diagnosis was, moreover, understood in a particular way. It was equated
with the *localization* of the seat of a disease: "To recognize diseases and
their seat is the most essential aspect of our art."[59] The attempt to realize
this ideal in clinical practice led to the creation of a distinctive genre of
case history that was essential to later aphasia studies.

Losing the Self

A prominent feature of Lordat's case histories was their polyphonic character: they accommodated the voices of several actors with no perceived
need to establish the predominance of any one; there was, in other words,
no fixed single perspective. Lordat figures in these narratives as one of a
number of characters. There is a genuine dialogue between him and those
whose ills he is called upon to treat. What is notable is not merely the
egalitarian relations that obtain between doctor and patient, but also the
complete visiblity of the former within the narrative. Lordat's status is
straightforward; his entrance upon the scene is clearly marked and brings
with it a shift in perspective. He is one of a number of empirical narrators
whose combined testimony effects the story.

In case histories of a slightly earlier epoch the medical self is still more
apparent and a good deal less modest. In the clinical observations of Marc-
Antoine Petit, for example, the surgeon is the protagonist of the narrative
which is predominantly told from his sometimes impressionistic viewpoint: thus when on one occasion applying the trepan Petit notes how "I
fell into a void formed by the separation of two tables."[60] Nor did Petit
hesitate to place his case reports in an autobiographical context where clinical detail is interwoven with his perception of historical events such as
the siege of Lyon. Rose Lépine, he noted, a patient at the Hôtel-Dieu of
that city, was wounded a second time by a bomb "hurled along with a
hundred others in one night on that asylum of humanity." This occurred
at 1 a.m. on the 26 August 1793; and "although the accident was serious
and required urgent attention, we could not provide her with the care she

[59] Ibid., p. 169.
[60] Marc-Antoine Petit, *Collection d'observations cliniques* (Lyon: Amable Leroy, 1815),
p. 285.

needed at a time when, in order to escape the fire of a cruel enemy, it was necessary precipitously to move a great distance the seat of one of France's finest hospitals."[61]

The identity of the narrator in Bouillaud's case histories is, in contrast, deeply problematic. This was no personal idiosyncracy of his way of writing; rather it reflected a genre bias found also in the case histories of his contemporaries. Within these narratives there is a striking reluctance to admit the presence of the self. This effacement is all the more remarkable when the intensely competitive and individualistic nature of Paris medicine is recalled. Although doctors were extremely anxious to take credit for discoveries, the form of the linguistic technologies employed to substantiate their knowledge claims conspired to conceal their role as historical actors.

On occasion medical authors expatiated upon the precautions they had taken to exclude the self from the process whereby "observations" were transformed by a process of inscription and reinscription into "facts." Léon Rostan (1791?–1866), for instance, claimed that:

> In order to avoid giving to my observations the colour of my way of thinking, I have not wished to collect them myself; I have entrusted them to intelligent students, who are trained and experienced, preferring to risk the loss of a few [observations] which might have been useful to me in the tableau I wished to trace rather than incur the suspicion of having bent the truth. My respect for [truth] has even been taken to the point where I have refrained from interfering with the drafting of observations; I have merely corrected a few stylistic faults that have escaped their authors.[62]

On this view the self represents a possible source of distortion that must be rigorously excluded from the process of composition if error was to be avoided. The question then arises of to whom or what does truth present itself if not to an empirical self? The answer appears to be to an absolute subjectivity that somehow transcends the contingent consciousness of any individual, but which exercises supervision and sovereignty over a world of objects.[63] The form of this genre of case history therefore lays claim to *objectivity*; the facts it presents are those that would be perceived by any

[61] Ibid., pp. 291–292.

[62] Léon Rostan, *Recherches sur le ramollissement du cerveau; ouvrage dans lequel on s'efforce de distinguer les diverses affections de ce viscère par des signes caractéristiques*, 2nd ed., (Paris: Béchet, 1823), pp. 3–4.

[63] For the Cartesian roots of this concept of the subject see: Dalai Judovitz, *Subjectivity and Representation in Descartes: The Origins of Modernity* (Cambridge: Cambridge University Press, 1988).

rational individual present during these events. The identity of the historical author is strictly incidental.[64]

Examination of Rostan's case histories themselves raises the related question of the identity of the narrator. What is clear is that a single voice dominates Rostan's case histories: they are, to use Bakhtin's term, examples of monologic rather than dialogic narrative.[65] These narratives manifest a reluctance to concede the existence of separate points of view within them; the perspectives of all the actors tend to be subsumed by that of the narrative voice.

This narrator arrogates properties to itself incompatible with the consciousness of any empirical self. It is evidently a fictive entity akin to the omniscient narrator of a novel;[66] yet the enigmatic nature of this subject is effectively obscured by a variety of conventional narrative devices. The interest and intent of the narrator is, however, undisguised: it seeks to derive a moral from the story recounted that is applicable to some scientific problematic. To return to the analogy with pictorial representation, the narrative voice is the textual equivalent of the Albertian disembodied eye. It imposes a single, dispassionate perspective on case history. In some ways, indeed, it imposes an annulment of narrative, striving to produce a *picture* of the case free from all accidental detail and the contingencies of history.[67]

These characteristics can be best displayed through an example of the genre. The LI° Observation, collected, Rostan notes, by M. Lembert, begins with the following passage:

> Madam Poteau, aged 75, of a robust constitution and of a sanguine temperament, had always had regular periods. The menopause had not been marked by any mishap; and this woman, very remarkable for gaiety and sagacity, had until a very advanced age enjoyed the best of health.[68]

This might seem an unremarkable preamble simply setting the scene for the case report proper. Most of the information it contains must have derived from the patient: who else would know the details, for example,

[64] On the aspirations of the emergent case history to the status of objective truth see: Susan C. Lawrence, *Charitable Knowledge: Hospital Pupils and Practitioners in Eighteenth-Century London* (Cambridge: Cambridge University Press, 1996), pp. 313–14, 341.

[65] Mikhail Bakhtin, *Problems of Dostoevsky's Poetics*, trans. Caryl Emerson (Manchester: Manchester Univ. Press, 1984), p. 7.

[66] Conversely, Lawrence Rothfield has argued that the narrator of the nineteenth-century novel exercises a form of medical panopticism: *Vital Signs: Medical Realism in Nineteenth-Century Fiction* (Princeton: Princeton University Press, 1992), especially p. 40.

[67] Martin Jay, *Downcast Eyes: The Denigration of Vision in Twentieth-Century French Thought* (Berkeley: University of California Press, 1994), pp. 61–63. Jay notes that much of the success of rational perspective can be attributed to its affinities with the new scientific world-view.

[68] Rostan, *Recherches*, p. 258.

of her menstrual history? But no attempt is made to attribute these facts to their source; they are blandly presented as part of the information immediately available to the narrative voice.

The process of disappropriation is furthered by the casual interweaving of what might once have been the patient's narrative with other matter: the fact that Madam Poteau is "very remarkable for her gaiety and sagacity" is one attributable to an external witness to the woman's nature. This tendency to interweave voices achieves a homogenizing effect; regardless of the actual source of these details, they are all represented as percepts of the narrator.

This process is reinforced in the clinical history proper. In December 1822 Poteau "suddenly lost consciousness, and was carried to the infirmary with a slight numbness of the limbs."[69] Here a single sentence combines testimony drawn from at least two sources in a seamless narrative texture. Who is the witness to the fact that the patient's loss of consciousness was sudden? Perhaps it was Poteau herself, perhaps a bystander. The information on the manner of her arrival at the infirmary cannot be ascribed to the patient; only she, however, could know of the lack of feeling in her arms and legs.

There is, in short, a powerful totalizing impulse at work in this narrative. The particularity of other voices is suppressed to create the fiction of a succession of events occurring within the ambit of a single observer. The qualitative differences between these events—the fact, for instance, that some relate to subjective states rather than objective occurrences—are treated with the same indifference.

Once within the infirmary Poteau becomes unequivocally the object of the medical gaze. But here too the narrator's knowledge exceeds that of an empirical observer. It is aware not only of the fact that the patient's speech is impaired but also knows that she, nonetheless, remained conscious of her state. Poteau's diseased speech is observed with a clinical detachment that gives no attention to the phenomenological aspects of the condition. After various verbal tests designed to elucidate the nature of the patient's speech lesion, "I concluded . . . that [her] condition did not depend solely upon verbal amnesia, but rather from the sudden and complete miscarriage of the memory for ideas and words."[70] If all these nuances are so negligible, what *does* matter to this narrator? The answer is that all of the details already mentioned, and even the observations of the patient's condition and treatment within the clinic represent merely a superficial and provisional account of the case. Their chief service is to adumbrate a more profound and compelling narrative.

[69] Ibid.
[70] Ibid., p. 259.

The contrast between the surface and the depths of the case can best be illustrated by juxtaposing two passages:

> Madame Poteau indicated that she experiences no pain in the head, but a general numbness. . . . Everything around the patient seemed to her to be in a continual spin. She was sometimes delirious, [but] more usually she was sufficiently rational, but her phrases were always incomplete.
>
> M. Rostan presumed that an inflammation of the meninges might exist.[71]

All Poteau's symptoms—including her sensations and impaired speech—signified only as clues for what might be going on inside her skull. This reality was accessible only to the clinician and served as an *explanation* for what had gone before.

This master narrative could, however, only be fully read after death; the autopsy was the true climax of the case history: all that went before was merely prologue. These autopsy reports are, moreover, not legitimated in terms of their alleged humanitarian value. There is no attempt to link the lesions discovered with the subject's way of life with a view to taking preventative measures.[72] These documents stand as tributes not to humanity but to the ideal of science.

The causes of what has befallen Madam Poteau are of no consequence to the narrator: what matters is what can be added to the stock of medical knowledge from an examination of the inside of her body. An outline of the postmortem findings is followed by reflection upon their meaning. Even though

> the considerations we have just read are of the highest interest; although they are founded upon an incontestable principle, namely, that the same organ cannot perform two different functions at the same time, . . . nevertheless, as there exist among the facts already observed some contradictory cases, I believe that it is prudent to multiply researches of this type to confirm these propositions or if necessary to qualify them; in either case this will be a conquest for truth, for which one should sacrifice everything.[73]

This genre of case history thus proclaims a moral imperative: the need for further work along similar lines. It contains code for the reproduction and growth of the genre.

Not all the cases recorded by Rostan show the same degree of narrative totalization. In some a plurality of voices, among which the medical is but

---

[71] Ibid., p. 260. In the original the second quotation follows on directly from the first.

[72] See: Thomas W. Laqueur, "Bodies, Details, and the Humanitarian Narrative," in *The New Cultural History*, ed. Lynn Hunt (Berkeley: Univ. of California Press, 1989), 176–204, esp. p. 178.

[73] Rostan, *Recherches*, pp. 263–264.

one, seems to be tolerated. Anne Marseille, for example, was struck down after she "received a most mortifying insult from one of the companions." A doctor is called to her, and his observations are recorded as those of an empirical observer. He orders a bleeding whereupon "speech returned almost immediately; the patient made use of it to express the relief that she felt."[74] But even when the patient is allowed a voice, this concession is limited by the hierarchy that clearly exists between the different contributions to the narrative. The patient's contribution is ascribed a lowly position within this order; it therefore becomes a suitable object for irony and for interpretative penetration by the narrator.[75] The final word belongs to Rostan who

> thought that the original symptoms were the result of a violent congestion of blood in the brain; that this congestion could have been more marked on one side than on the other; that indeed a slight sanguinous discharge had formed in the right hemisphere, and that this explained why the symptoms were after a few days confined to the left side of the body.[76]

This occult sequence of events available only to the clinician constitutes the true meaning or moral of the case.

Even if the patient's narrative does not "disappear," it can still be drained of significance.[77] The narrative of Thérèse Chérame commences with the patient's reported speech:

> During the night of Tuesday to Wednesday last, she dreamed that a madwoman chased her, caught her and cut her throat; the pain of this imaginary torment drew cries from her that woke her companions.

Chérame awoke in a sweat, but her terror soon dissipated and she once more fell asleep. When in the morning she attempted to get out of bed, however, Chérame found her lower limbs were paralyzed. This episode is necessarily recounted from the patient's perspective—we are told that she felt pain in her legs which was worse on the left side—but this perspective is fully engrossed by the narrator's consciousness.[78]

---

[74] Ibid., pp. 293–294.

[75] Compare the discussion of the various degrees of integrity allowed to differently ranked forms of reported speech in: Valentin Nikolaevic Volosinov, *Marxism and the Philosophy of Language*, trans. Ladislav Matejka and I. R. Titunik (New York: Seminar Press, 1973), pp. 119–23.

[76] Rostan, *Recherches*, p. 295.

[77] On the diminished significance of patients' own accounts of their illness see: Mary E. Fissell, "The Disappearance of the Patient's Narrative and the Invention of Hospital Medicine," in *British Medicine in an Age of Reform*, ed. Roger French and Andrew Wear (London: Routledge, 1991), pp. 92–109.

[78] Rostan, *Recherches*, pp. 433–434.

Thereafter the narrative is monopolized by the medical voice. The patient's symptoms are analyzed and those deemed essential are differentiated from the accidental; what is of interest is not the illness as a whole, but the "principal disease." The nature of the lesion that might be responsible for the loss of movement in the lower limbs is then projected.[79]

The account of the dream, to which Chérame presumably attached some significance in her own account of the inception of her illness, is thus left dangling within the overall narrative. It is, at most, accorded the status of a curiosity with no import for the understanding of the case. The inclusion of this detail serves only to reinforce the omniscience of the narrative voice: it encompasses even the secrets of the patient's sleep.[80]

Legislating for Speech

The outstanding genre features of Rostan's case histories are also evident in Bouillaud's narratives. Indeed, the latter drew upon the former's cases freely for material with which to substantiate his points. Although they might differ on details of doctrine (Rostan was to repudiate Bouillaud's putative localization of speech), they inhabited the same linguistic universe of clinical discourse. Consequently there were no translation difficulties to be overcome; through the medium of a shared way of writing particular instances had become a universal resource. The clinical experience of each individual involved in generating these texts was now available to all participants in the game.

Bouillaud began his "Recherches cliniques" seemingly some distance from the subject of speech and its impediments. His avowed aim was to combat the views put forward by Pierre Flourens (1794–1867) in his *Recherches expérimentales sur les propriétés du système nerveux*.[81] Specifically, Bouillaud wished to discredit Flourens' doctrine that the cerebral hemispheres played no part in locomotor functions. The paper was thus at once locked into a dialectic with an unequivocally physiological text, both documents purporting to establish general truths about the part played by the brain in the life of the organism.

---

[79] Ibid., pp. 434–435.

[80] All the patients in the cases discussed are female. A hospital patient's sex did not, however, determine the way in which he or she was represented in the record; male patients were subjected to similar treatment.

[81] Pierre Flourens, *Recherches expérimentales sur les propriétés et les fonctions du système nerveux, dans les animaux vertébrés* (Paris: Crevot, 1824). Flourens was by this time also a vehement opponent of Gall's doctrine of organology. See: Edwin Clarke and L. S. Jacyna, *Nineteenth-Century Origins of Neuroscientific Concepts* (Berkeley: University of California Press, 1987), pp. 267–68.

But whereas Flourens had inferred his conclusions from animal experiments, Bouillaud's laboratory was the clinic. Any practitioner at all familiar with clinical inquiries, he asserted, would have observed many cases where cerebral lesions had impaired the motor functions. For Bouillaud, however, it was "not enough to know in a general manner that the cerebrum is indispensable for the production of various muscular movements; there is still the question of determining whether the different parts that make up the cerebrum do not each have particular movements under their control."[82] The complex premises underpinning the assumption that these were legitimate, indeed necessary, questions are simply elided.

Bouillaud cited various previous authors who had claimed that it was possible to distinguish between the parts of the brain that innervated particular limbs. But it was an error "to believe that the limbs are the only parts for the movements of which there exist particular cerebral centres." In fact, *all* movements which were "under the empire of intelligence" were regulated by such a center. Bouillaud proposed to confine himself, however, to one such class of movement: those involved in articulate speech.[83] By analogy speech too must have its "special center."

The fact that Bouillaud chose to categorize speech as a form of motor phenomenon is itself a point of some significance; but one which will not be developed here. Instead the above remarks are intended to provide a context for the use made of clinical histories in the "Recherches cliniques" and in Bouillaud's other discussions of the anatomical relations of speech. These narratives were recounted in order to vindicate a theoretic position; the characters who people these accounts are therefore stripped of all attributes other than those seen to further this end.

Bouillaud subdivided his theory into a number of subordinate propositions for the truth of each of which a number of cases was supposed to testify. He first attempted to prove that there was, indeed, "a cerebral nervous centre devoted to the organs of speech." Catherine Thirion, a forty-four year old of a "nervous-sanguine" constitution, was an unwitting witness to this fact:

> on the 10 December 1822 she suddenly lost her voice, and some time later made her way to the hôpital Cochin. She heard and understood perfectly everything that was said to her, but was unable to utter the least word. She expressed her ideas clearly by means of writing, and advised us in this manner that she had a pain in the forehead, etc. Annoyed by her muteness, she grew impatient, gesticulated vigorously, and wept. Following a copious bleeding, this woman recovered the full use of her speech after a few days.[84]

[82] Bouillaud, "Recherches," pp. 25–26.
[83] Ibid., p. 27.
[84] Ibid., p. 28.

This narrative is notable for its unified perspective. The onset of Thirion's illness and her eventual progress to the hospital, as well as her subsequent condition, are all visible from a single viewpoint. As a case Thirion moreover exists solely to make Bouillaud's point. We are told that in her written communications she complained of headache; but this serves to prove that only her capacity for spoken language was affected. The irritation and misery engendered by her condition are reported; these affective details demonstrate, however, the overall integrity of her mental faculties. Once she recovers her speech Thirion is dismissed from the text as of no further interest.

This along with two other cases sufficed to prove that "paralysis of the organs of speech can occur in isolation independent of all other paralysis." It was therefore necessary to assume the existence of an entity that might account for this phenomenon: within the brain there must be an organ "devoted to the regulation, to the *coordination* of the marvellous movements by which man through the use of his voice communicates his thoughts, expresses his feelings, and, so to speak, depicts the movements of his soul." Bouillaud called this entity "the legislative organ of speech."[85] This organ, rather than any of the human actors, is the true protagonist of the narrative.

According to the organicist canon it was, however, necessary to go further and to localize this organ within the brain. Bouillaud's second proposition was therefore that "the cerebral nervous centre presiding over the movement of the organs of speech has its seat in the anterior lobes of the brain." The facts made this claim incontrovertible. These "facts" comprised three additional cases, two of which had ended in death followed by autopsy, while one Bouillaud had been fortunate enough to cure.[86] Only the first two provided conclusive evidence; the third case was, from this point of view, unsatisfactory because only conjectural conclusions could be derived from it.[87] It went without saying that direct observation of the diseased brain after death alone constituted sufficient evidence.

These case histories are inserted into a narrative of discovery: Bouillaud's account of how he came to the conclusions now embodied in the text. After his own observations had suggested the possibility that there existed "an intimate relationship between the more or less absolute loss

---

[85] Ibid., pp. 29–30.

[86] "Quant au sujet de la troisième de nos précédentes observations, comme nous eûmes le bonheur de le guérir, je ne le donnerai ici comme favorable à notre opinion que par analogie." Ibid., p. 31. The passage is notable for the rare gesture towards humanitarian sentiment that it contains.

[87] Ibid., pp. 30–31.

of speech and a more or less profound alteration in the anterior lobes of the brain," he sought to substantiate this hypothesis by reference to the cases of other observers. He had no difficulty in finding such confirmation in the published works of Rostan and others; but was surprised that it had not "entered into the spirit of these excellent observers to make the easy discovery" that had instead fallen to Bouillaud.[88]

Bouillaud was thus engaged in a simultaneous process of alienation and appropriation. On the one hand, he tried to enhance the credibility of his assertions by adducing observations recorded by others. He therefore seemed to reduce his own role in the compositional process. Such show of objectivity and of elision of the self conformed to the genre biases already noted. On the other hand, Bouillaud subtly but emphatically asserted his own title to scientific originality. Disciplinary restraints were thus subject to subtle forms of subversion and circumvention. Bouillaud's argumentative strategy was served by implying a distinction between the "writer" who merely inscribed a history and the "author" to whom credit for the full understanding of the import of that description belonged.[89]

Some of the cases that Bouillaud adduced were "positive" in their import—they demonstrated the connection between lesions of the frontal regions of the brain and speech loss. These were complemented by "negative" instances where lesions of different parts of the brain were accompanied by other symptoms while language capacity remained intact. Taken together these numerous cases were more than sufficient to demonstrate the validity of Bouillaud's thesis: "How can one hereafter dispute this truth [which] we have established by experience and by observation[?]"[90]

The establishment of this "truth" was unequivocally the object of the text. The narratives of disease embodied within it were wholly subordinate to this aim; and the individuals contained in those histories—patients and doctors alike—existed merely as "witnesses" to a truth manifest in but which transcended the particularities of any case. The various patients who figured in these "Recherches Cliniques" did not exist as concrete individuals but merely as ciphers for a universal "man." The illnesses that beset them were conceptualized not as lesions of a particular self but as exercises whereby nature elucidated for the edification of science the "great faculty by which man is distinguished among all the animals."[91]

[88] Ibid., p. 34.
[89] See the distinction between author, writer, and narrator in: Dominick LaCapra, *"Madame Bovary" on Trial* (Ithaca: Cornell Univ. Press, 1982), p. 63.
[90] Bouillaud, "Recherches," p. 40.
[91] Ibid., p. 43.

Conclusion

The case histories Bouillaud supplied in the "Recherches cliniques" are terse to the point of minimalism. The cases he recounted in his later publications—notably in his treatise on encephalitis—tended to be more expansive. While the former provide special insight into the system of subordination to which clinical observations were subject within his overall project, the latter give a fuller insight into the status accorded to the patient within this textual regime.

As in his address to the Académie Royale de la Médecine, Bouillaud drew upon various sources for histories reproduced in the *Traité clinique*; there is, in consequence, some variety in the style and content of the narratives found there. Nor was he solely concerned with cases in which speech was affected. Nonetheless, those case histories that do deal with language loss exhibit the genre characteristics already noted. There is a tendency towards a totalized narrative in which all other voices are subordinated to that of a dominant engrossing subject. The biographical details of a patient called "Maintion" are reported in unusual detail: although now a house painter, he had previously been a soldier. He had left the army six years before, but had arrived in Paris only two months before his admission to the hospital. All this might be taken as Maintion's own account of himself. But when the preamble goes on, without any change in register, to record that "For two years he had shown signs of imbecility and a complete loss of memory," and that while a soldier he had at times "presented" symptoms of mental derangement, the patient has ceased to speak for himself and has become the object of another's narrative. Who that other might be is unexplicated.[92]

In these accounts the patient's narrative autonomy is reduced to an occasional "dit-elle." When the patient's words do appear in the form of reported speech, they tend to be infiltrated and editorialized by the authorial voice in ways that modify the import that the reader attaches to these utterances. For instance, "the [patient's] ideas are more confused; the patient did not say he was in pain. . . . His condition was improved, as he said himself."[93]

The extraclinical existence of the patient is usually accorded, at most, a perfunctory mention as if the whole purpose of his or her life was to become ill so as to qualify as an object of medical attention. Thus the identity of a seventy-four-year-old man struck down with paralysis is

---

[92] Bouillaud, *Traité*, pp. 85–86. In some of the case histories there is an identification of the source of the patient's impressions recorded, e.g., ibid., p. 101. These are, however, best viewed as imperfectly edited approximations to the typical clinical narrative of this genre.

[93] Ibid., p. 82.

compressed to: "Clérin, gardener, recently afflicted with apoplexy at which time he entered hospital."[94] Once admitted Clérin becomes an object of contemplation: "Immobility, stupor, general numbness, loss of speech, hearing very dull, deviation of the mouth to the left."[95] The affection of speech is embedded within a wider pathological picture; the notion that this might be a symptom with special significance for the patient does not occur.

But the medical gaze is not restricted to the patient's external appearance and performances; it is capable of penetrating into his or her consciousness. The narrator knows, for instance, that "when the patient was alone and left to himself his physiognomy was sad and dejected." When, however,

> during the visit he was surrounded [by others] and stimulated, either by talk or by pinches, he was aware of jokes; in his eyes, in his countenance [*figure*] were etched all the emotions of his soul.[96]

Shortly before Clérin's death these emotions turned to sadness. His demise marks, however, an abrupt change in the narrative register: "Before the autopsy, M. Serres announced the nature of the malady." In short, the real essence of the events under consideration is about to be revealed. "Let us now try," Bouillaud proposed, "to determine the portion of the brain to the lesion of which corresponds the loss of speech and the paralysis of the muscles necessary to the production of this important phenomenon." This was as "interesting" a question from a physiological as from a clinical viewpoint.[97] The briefly realized pathos of Clérin's predicament therefore gives way to the pursuit of scientific goals.

This chapter has not attempted a revision of Bouillaud's position within the existing historiography of aphasia studies. It has instead drawn attention to the linguistic technology with which his texts obtained their effects. This technology was not peculiar to Bouillaud nor his invention, but derived from a culture in which a certain genre of medical writing was already firmly established. This genre lent itself to the production of certain ends while remaining oblivious to others; it was, in particular, well adapted to the recruitment of a homogenized clinical material to the project of a scientific medicine.

Nor have I attempted to show that Lordat is an "unjustly neglected" figure in need of rehabilitation: from the point of view of the dominant Western medical tradition his neglect is perfectly just. A study of his ac-

[94] Ibid., p. 156.
[95] Ibid.
[96] Ibid., pp. 156–157.
[97] Ibid., pp. 157–158.

counts of language loss does, however, serve to highlight the artifactual nature of what became the received version of the neurological case history. The latter is revealed not as natural and comprehensive but as a highly contrived and selective form of narrative. Much of what might be said is excluded; while what *is* said is articulated in a very particular form.

The form that the generic case history took was, as has been noted, determined by the kinds of language certified by the nineteenth-century clinic. More generally, it bore a strong resemblance to forms of writing that became dominant in the natural sciences around the same period. In particular, the effacement of the personal identity of the author evident in these texts with its concomitant claim of objectivity was also typical of the characteristic mode of the emergent modern scientific research report.[98]

Medical discourse about language and its loss could, in short, have taken a different form. Just how different may be illustrated by a final case history drawn from the writings of John Hennen, a contemporary British surgeon:

> CAPTAIN B—, a particular friend of mine, was wounded by a musket-ball in the head at Waterloo on the 18th June [1815]. On the 19th he was brought into the city of Brussels in charge of a medical officer, who gave me a most melancholy account of his case. On approaching the waggon in which he was conveyed, I was insensibly attracted to that part of it where he was stretched, by a low protracted moan, as of a person in extreme pain, but very weak. On calling him by name, he sat up, caught me by the hand, which he kissed most fervently, pointed to his head, and then to the site of a former wound which he had received at the storming of Badajos, from the effects of which I had the good fortune to relieve him. He then burst into tears, but without the power of uttering a distinct word.[99]

His other duties notwithstanding Hennen maintained contact with this patient and monitored his progress. On one such visit,

> he grasped my hand with great fervour, looked piteously into my face, and, to my inquiries as to his feelings, he uttered the monosyllable "THER," to which in the course of the day, he added "O;" and for the three next days, whenever addressed, he slowly, distinctly, and in the most pathetic tone, repeated the words, "O;THER: O;THER:" as if to prove his powers of pronunciation. . . . I therefore resolved to write to his family, and, before doing so, I printed in large characters on a sheet of paper the following words, "SHALL

[98] Gyorgy Markus, "Why Is There No Hermeneutics of Natural Sciences? Some Preliminary Theses," *Science in Context* 1 (1987): 5–51, especially pp. 12–13.

[99] John Hennen, *Principles of Military Surgery, Comprising Observations on the Arrangement, Police, and Practice of Hospitals, and on the History, Treatment, and Anomalies of Variola and Syphilis* (Edinburgh: Archibald Constable, 1820), pp. 305–6.

I WRITE TO YOUR MOTHER?" that being the wish which it appeared to me he so long and ardently had laboured to utter. It is impossible to describe the illumination of his countenance on reading these talismanic words; he grasped and pressed my hand with warmth, burst into tears, and gave every demonstration of having obtained the boon which he had endeavoured to solicit.[100]

It is unnecessary to belabor the ways in which this narrative differs from Bouillaud's histories of language loss. As with Lordat, there is a determination to present the condition as a lesion of a developed historical individual with whom the practitioner has a complex relationship. What is also striking are the motifs of empathy and gratitude that recur throughout the narrative. Conversely, there is an absence of any physio-pathological context for the case: what matters is the particular instant not the general principles that this patient may exemplify.

The question of why a particular genre of medical writing became dominant to the virtual exclusion of other renderings of clinical reality cannot be answered solely by reference to linguistic conventions. Language acts form only one aspect of the totality of a discourse; the form of the social relations within which linguistic conventions are developed must also be taken into account. Bouillaud's case histories approximate most closely to paradigmatic notions of a clinical record because they originated in the paradigmatic institution of modern medicine: the public hospital conceived as a place where teaching and research were privileged activities.[101] There was, moreover, an important *quantitative* difference between hospital and private practice: the former could provide the practitioner with far more instances of a particular complaint. The literary apparatus outlined above was a technology for managing this multiplicity and rendering it of service. One corollary of this process of inscription was that these patients lost much of their individuality; they became part of a *series*. The due registration of this series in turn made it possibile to create an archive that could be exploited in the name of science (see chapter 3).

The reified notion of the patient that these texts embody is also a faithful reflection of the lack of power of those committed to those establishments; in return for this charity, the patient had effectively surrendered the right to be considered as a self.[102] These "were the terms of the contract by

---

[100] Ibid., p. 308.

[101] For an account of the introduction of these new priorities into the Parisian hospitals in the aftermath of the Revolution see: Dora B. Weiner, *The Citizen-Patient in Revolutionary and Imperial Paris* (Baltimore: Johns Hopkins University Press, 1993), pp. 149–51.

[102] In the rare instance where a patient is ascribed something approximating to selfhood, he is significantly of a higher social status than the common hospital patient. See the case of "Captain Thavernier": Bouillaud, *Traité*, pp. 125–127. Cf. the case of the "militaire" recorded on pp. 128–129.

which rich and poor participated in the organization of clinical experience. . . . [T]he clinic . . . is the *interest* paid by the poor on the capital
that the rich have consented to invest in the hospital."[103]

An analysis of the forms of medical writing that flourished in that nidus
can, however, illuminate what is most basic to the cognitive processes of
modern medicine. An exposition of the narrative artifices of the case history can, in particular, help make vocal the "tacit form of violence, all the
more abusive for its silence,"[104] inherent in a medicine that recounts in
order to teach or learn rather than to heal. The hope that these investigations might lead to effective therapy was never abandoned; it was, however,
deferred.

[103] Michel Foucault, *The Birth of the Clinic: An Archaeology of Medical Perception*, trans.
A. M. Sheridan Smith (London: Tavistock Publications, 1973), p. 85.

[104] Ibid., p. 84.

TWO

"THE WORD TURNED UPSIDE DOWN"

I N *THE ORDER OF THINGS* Michel Foucault describes how in the nineteenth century language ceased to be the transparent vehicle of knowledge and became itself an object of investigation.[1] Foucault had in mind the emergence during this period of a science of linguistics which viewed language as an object with its own structure and history—as an entity independent of the human subjects that articulate it. The nineteenth century, however, also witnessed the emergence of another body of knowledge specifically concerned with linguistic performance, or its absence.

This other science of language was elaborated in the clinic. It was a medical discourse primarily concerned with the perturbations of language. It was a received medical dictum, however, that disease can illuminate the normal; the pathology of language was accordingly recruited to elucidate its physiology. The medical discourse of language possessed a particular form and orientation: it sought to establish the ultimate conditions of language use. It located these conditions not in grammar or logic but in the body. This was not in itself a novelty—the existence of "vocal organs" had been acknowledged long before the nineteenth century. What distinguished nineteenth-century medicine was its insistence that the tongue and larynx were only proximate instruments of speech; the ultimate physical substrate of language lay in the brain.

It is unusually easy to specify the inception of this claim. In 1825 Jean-Baptiste Bouillaud proposed that the "legislative organ" of language was located in the frontal lobes of the brain[2] (see chapter 1). Although he gave due credit to Franz Josef Gall's claim to have anticipated this finding, Bouillaud is generally allowed the status of the founder of the neurophysiology of language. His early pronouncements on the subject proved, however, to be something of a false dawn. Bouillaud's claims attracted more

---

[1] Michel Foucault, *The Order of Things: An Archaeology of the Human Sciences* (London: Tavistock Publications, 1970), pp. 294–95.

[2] Jean-Baptiste Bouillaud, "Recherches cliniques propres à démontrer que la perte de la parole correspond à la lésion des lobules antérieurs du cerveau, et à confirmer l'opinion de M. GALL, sur le siège de l'organe du langage articulé," *Archive générales de médecine* 8 (1825): 25–45.

criticism than support; and by 1842 it was possible to conclude that other pathologists had "disputed and successfully controverted this opinion."[3]

In 1861 a more decisive event occurred. Paul Broca (1824–80), another French clinician and pathologist, propounded a more refined notion of the cerebral localization of language. According to him, the seat of language lay in the third frontal convolution of the brain—an area which eventually became known as "Broca's region." Broca's assertions also proved controversial. But in contrast to the fate that overtook Bouillaud's doctrines, this later promulgation of a theory of the cerebral localization of language attracted sufficient support not only to survive but to become orthodoxy.[4]

This is to take, as have most previous historians of the subject, an essentially constructive view of Bouillaud and Broca's "contributions" to nineteenth-century thought. Even those who are critical of particular aspects of their theories, acknowledge that they helped to lay the bases of a scientific understanding of the human faculty of language. If medical philology is regarded as a discreet discourse then this orientation towards Bouillaud's and Broca's writings is justified and indeed beyond dispute. But if these texts are considered in a more extensive context they acquire fresh significance.

I will argue that the adumbration of a physiological understanding of language was as much a destructive as a constructive operation. The mere articulation of the claim that such a discourse was possible challenged older understandings of the place of language in the order of things. It staked a claim for a naturalistic understanding of a uniquely significant area of human experience. Much of the opposition that these early essays aroused was derived from a more or less clear perception of the full cultural import of the content of these apparently abstruse and technical documents.

Word, Reason, Power

One way in which to address the negating, subversive aspects of these texts is, adapting Bakhtin's terms, to consider the early inquiry into the physiological conditions of language as a "grotesque symposium"—as foci

[3] G. J. Guthrie, *On Injuries of the Head affecting the Brain* (London: John Churchill, 1842), p. 46.

[4] In later publications Broca elaborated upon this initial claim arguing that the organ of language was represented unilaterally. See: Anne Harrington, *Medicine, Mind, and the Double Brain: A Study in Nineteenth-Century Thought* (Princeton: Princeton University Press, 1987), pp. 75–77.

at which processes of inversion, challenge, and transformation occur.[5] This is a matter both of style and substance. Ludic strategies are evident in these scientific texts where privileged objects are subjected to an irreverent scrutiny in which such devices as parody, caricature, and hyperbole are freely employed.[6] The overall effect of these linguistic modes is to erode established distinctions between the material and the spiritual, the profane and the sacred. Although in a sense "playful," these documents also epitomize forms of cultivated aggression: as Peter Gay has argued, in the nineteenth century even humor could serve the cause of cultural belligerence.[7] The nature of language, and in particular the issue of its status within the human constitution, became a site for such contestation because of the unique value that had over the centuries been invested in the Word.

In a passage from the *Génie du christianisme* (1802) François René de Chateaubriand invited his readers to contemplate

> a new-born child that a nurse holds in her arms. What has he said to give such joy to this old man, to this grown man, to this woman? Two or three half-formed syllables, which no-one understands: yet here are rational beings transported by joy, from the grandfather, who knows all about life, to the young mother who is still an innocent! Who then has endowed the word of man with such power? Why does the sound of a human voice move you so powerfully? What captivates you is a mystery that pertains to more elevated causes than the interest one might take in the age of this child: something tells you that these inarticulate words are the first stirrings of an immortal spirit [*pensée immortelle*].[8]

This somewhat lurid passage hints at some of the significance that has attached to the faculty of language in modern Western culture. Speech is conceived as something peculiarly distinctive of human nature. It was, moreover, a property that raised humans above the mundane realm and indicates their supernal character and destiny.

---

[5] See: Mikhail Bakhtin, *Rabelais and his World*, trans. Helene Iswolsky (Cambridge, Mass.: M.I.T. Press, 1968); idem, *Problems of Dostoevsky's Poetics*, trans. Caryl Emerson, (Manchester: Manchester University Press, 1984). Because of "carnival's" association, especially in Bakhtin's work, with specifically proletarian cultural forms, the concept of "symbolic inversion" as developed by Barbara Babcock may be more apposite: Barbara A. Babcock, *The Reversible World: Symbolic Inversion in Art and Society* (Ithaca: Cornell University Press, 1978), pp. 13–36.

[6] For a discussion of the presence of grotesque elements in Darwin's writings see: Donald Ulin, "A Clerisy of Worms in Darwin's Inverted World," *Victorian Studies*, 35 (1991–92): 295–308.

[7] Peter Gay, *The Cultivation of Hatred: The Bourgeois Experience Victorian to Freud Volume III* (London: Harper Collins, 1993), chapter 5.

[8] François René de Chateaubriand, *Génie du christianisme*, ed. Maurice Regard (Paris: Gallimard, 1978), p. 614.

The strong association between language and humanity had Cartesian roots. In the *Discours de la methode* Descartes argued that nothing obstructed a purely mechanistic notion of the actions of the animal body. Animals were merely automata contrived by the ingenuity of God; although vastly more complicated, they did not in essence differ from man-made machines. So much so that "if there were such machines which possessed the organs and the form of an ape or of any other irrational animal, we would have no way of knowing that they were not of entirely the same nature as these animals." A machine fashioned in the form of a man and capable of imitating his actions could, however, be infallibly distinguished by means of two tests,

> Of which the first is that they could never employ words or any other sign . . . as we do to express our thoughts to others. For we may easily conceive a machine so constructed that it emits words, and even that it utters some appropriate to the action of the material influences that cause a certain change in its organs . . . ; but not that it should arrange [words] in various ways in order to respond to the sense of all that is said in its presence, as even the most stupid men can do.[9]

The same test served to distinguish men not only from inanimate simulacra, but also from animals. It was, Descartes declared, most remarkable that there are "no men so dull and so stupid, not even the insane, that they are incapable of putting different words together, so as to compose a discourse through which they express their thoughts; and, on the other hand, there is no other animal, however perfect or wellborn it may be, that can do the same." This incapacity did not have an organic basis—animals were equipped with all the requisite organs for speech; the deficiency was intellectual. Their inability to speak proved "not only that animals have less reason than men, but that they have none at all."[10]

Speech was therefore not only the faculty whereby man distinguished himself from inanimate matter and from the animals; it was the prime token of the rational and spiritual aspect of his nature. In the words of a follower of Descartes, "speech is always composed of two elements: namely, the formation of the sound, which can only come from the body; and the meaning or the idea conjoined to the sound, which can only be derived from the soul."[11] The more he was convinced that some of the

[9] René Descartes, *Oeuvres de Descartes*, ed. Charles Adam and Paul Tannery, 11 vols in 13, (Paris: J. Vrin, 1973), vol. 6, pp. 56–57.

[10] Ibid., pp. 57–58.

[11] [Geraud] de Cordemoy, *Dissertations physiques sur le discernement du corps & de l'ame: sur la parole, et sur le système de Monsieur Descartes*, 3rd ed., 2 vols. (Paris: Veuve de Denis Nion, 1690), vol. 2, p. [vii].

bodies he observed in the world were capable of understanding his words and of making intelligible utterances of their own, the more the philosopher was assured that these beings possessed a soul akin to his own.[12]

This association between language, humanity, and reason persisted into the eighteenth and nineteenth century, as did the dualistic understanding of the mechanism of language acts. According to Nicolas Beauzée, "All *languages [langues]* have a common goal—the enunciation of thought. To achieve this all employ the same instrument, the voice: it is like the spirit and the body of language."[13] Within this dualist dynamic the bodily side of language was, moreover, unequivocally subordinate to the spiritual or intellectual aspect. It was this conception of language that Jacques Lordat articulated.

Antoine Court de Gébelin agreed that "speech is the depiction of our thoughts by means of the vocal instrument." He added that language was "the fundamental part of the human essence and glory, [which] distinguishes man from the other beings with which he shares the fruits of the earth and which have in common with him all the phenomena of animal life." All these other animate beings were capable of no more than an "inarticulate cry."[14] This unique faculty was, moreover, not of natural origins: "it is God who made of man a speaking being."[15]

This was to take a clear side in the eighteenth-century debate between those who argued that language was a human invention and those who maintained that it must be derived from God. In his exposition of the various theories on the origin of language that had been articulated in these debates Louis Gabriel Ambroise de Bonald emphasized how the stance adopted on this issue tended to reflect a much wider range of philosophical commitments. One school regarded language as a gift given to man by the power that formed his body and his other intellectual powers. Others—"happily few in number"—saw man as the product of the play of natural forces; they believed that he had evolved from more primitive forms of life and ultimately from brute matter. Mind and language had been acquired, like all other human attributes, in the course of time and thanks to "favourable circumstances." A third group sought to steer a course between these extremes; their explanation was accordingly "feeble and inconsequential like all *moderate* opinions in philosophy [*morale*]." They conceded that the world was the work of a supreme cause. This

---

[12] Ibid., pp. 7–8.

[13] Nicolas Beauzée, "Langue," in *Encyclopédie méthodique. Gramaire et littérature*, 3 vols., (Paris: Panckoucke, 1784), vol. 2, p. 410.

[14] [Antoine] Court de Gébelin, *Histoire naturelle de la parole, ou grammaire universelle à l'usage des jeunes gens*, 2nd ed. (Paris: Plancher, 1816), pp. 2–4.

[15] Ibid., p. 17.

power had endowed man with a general capacity for self-development to which could be ascribed the invention of language.[16]

These three opinions on the origin of language corresponded, Bonald held, to three different position on "the existence and nature of the first cause . . . : 1st theism which believes God the author of all . . . ; 2nd atheism which only admits matter or *nature* as a creative and conserving cause; 3rd deism which holds a middle ground between theism and atheism, recognizing a supreme being as the first cause of the universe, but refusing him the government and direction of man and of society."[17] The theist school insisted upon man's dependence upon God for the gift of language as for all else. Moreover, while theism saw mind and language as superimposed upon the animal part of human nature, the atheist saw the mental faculties, speech included, as evolving from corporeal properties.

Bonald himself had no doubt that "language was given to man, not invented by him."[18] The capacity merely to articulate words was not the crucial aspect of the phenomenon:

since this faculty also appears among some animals. It is the faculty of understanding [speech] when it strikes our ear, and of attaching an idea to it, which is the exclusive property of the human species and its most noble prerogative; for animals hear our speech without comprehending it, it is for them merely a sound, become by frequent repetition a material and sensible sign, inseparable from certain movements which one has taught them.[19]

It was, on the contrary, the capacity to "understand the expression of moral and incorporeal things which appears to be the distinctive quality [and] the special characteristic of human intelligence"; and it was this power that justified the claim that "the supreme intelligence made [man] in his own image."[20]

Language was thus invested with enormous significance and dignity. It was the:

light of the moral world . . . bond of society, life of intelligences, store of all truths, of all laws, of all happenings, speech rules man, orders society, explains the universe . . . it is the profoundest mystery of our being, and far from having been capable of inventing it, man cannot even understand it.[21]

---

[16] Louis Gabriel Ambroise de Bonald, *Recherches philosophiques sur les premiers objets des connoissances morales*, 3rd ed., 2 vols. (Paris: Adrien le Clere, 1838), vol. 1, pp. 121–122.

[17] Ibid., p. 123.

[18] Ibid., p. 171.

[19] Ibid., p. 201.

[20] Ibid., pp. 201–202.

[21] Ibid., p. 142.

The final attribute of incomprehensibility is especially important: language was, like life, something which man enjoyed but which eluded all efforts at explanation.

The inscrutability thus attributed to language posed a problem for the early exponents of philology.[22] Ernest Renan sought to maintain the mystique of the subject while arguing that there was nonetheless scope for investigation and discovery. The origins of language, he conceded, would always "remain mysterious." But it was possible to surmise "to which order of facts one needs to refer it and from what order of conceptions it is proper to deduce it."[23]

The order of conceptions to which Renan drew special attention were those derived from biological science; indeed, rightly conceived, philology was itself "one of the life sciences." It was neccessary to consider language as "an organic whole, endowed with an intrinsic vitality." The "vegetation" of each family of languages proceeded according to the same uniform laws.[24] These laws were essentially those of ontogenesis as revealed by the science of embryology: languages were to be situated unequivocally "in the category of living things."[25]

From this perspective the antitheses of the eighteenth-century debate on the origins of language seemed crude and false, and Bonald's contributions were dismissed as of the same ilk.[26] According to Renan language was neither an invention of humanity nor a God-given gift:

the need to express his ideas and feelings is natural to man . . . There is nothing arbitrary in the use of articulation as a sign of thought. It is neither because of suitability or of convenience, nor by imitation of animals, that man has chosen speech to formulate and communicate his ideas, but rather because speech is natural to him, both in respect of its organic production and in respect of its expressive value.[27]

Renan therefore seemed to incline towards a naturalistic concept of the faculty of language. He compared it with *other* bodily functions such as vision and hearing.[28] At the same time, however, he took pains to preserve

---

[22] For the early history of linguistics see: Hans Aarsleff, *From Locke to Saussure: Essays on the Study of Language and Intellectual History* (London: Athlone Press, 1982); idem, *The Study of Language in England 1780–1860* (London: Athlone Press, 1983); R. H. Robins, *A Short History of Linguistics* (London: Longman, 1967); R. Harris and T. J. Taylor, *Landmarks in Linguistic Thought: The Western Tradition from Socrates to Saussure* (London: Routledge, 1989).

[23] Ernst Renan, *De l'origine du langage* (Paris: Michel, Lévy, Frères, 1858), pp. 87–88.

[24] Ibid., pp. 86–87.

[25] Ibid., p. 187.

[26] Ibid., p. 87.

[27] Ibid., pp. 89–90.

[28] Ibid., p. 90.

the association of language with the "higher" aspects of human nature; language was, he declared, "the expressive form and outer garment of thought." He wished, moreover, to temper his seemingly mundane view of the nature of speech with a continued recognition that the faculty possessed a transcendent aspect:

> on the one hand, speech is the work of man and of the forces inherent in him; on the other, there is nothing reflective, nothing artificially contrived in language, no more than in the mind [*esprit*]. All there is is the work of forces intrinsic to human nature, acting without consciousness and as if under the active influence of the divinity.[29]

The true author of the "spontaneous products of consciousness" might therefore be conceived either as "human nature or . . . the superior cause of nature. At this limit, it is a matter of indifference whether to attribute the causality to God or to man."[30]

The constraints upon Renan's readiness to divest language of its mystique were apparent in his discussion of Karl Ferdinand Becker's "organicist" notion of the mechanisms of speech. Becker had maintained that "the action [*Verrichtung*] of speech is an organic action." By this he meant that speech *"emerges with an inner necessity from the organic life of men."*[31] Taken in isolation this might be taken for a crudely materialist understanding of language. In fact, Becker depicted spirit and matter as two aspects of a unitary reality. It was a general law of living nature that "every activity becomes manifest in a material substance, every psychic phenomenon [*Geistige*] in a bodily form [*Leiblichen*]."[32]

The particular corporeal embodiment of the spiritual activity of language was "the word." Whether it was actually articulated or merely imagined, "the word is the natural body of the concept."[33] In other words, "just as the eye is the organ for the natural function of vision, so is language the organ for what is for man the equally natural function of representing and communicating thought." This was a monistic rather than a dualistic understanding both of human nature generally and of language in particular: "in the same way that man is a unity of spirit and body, so the word is a unity of concept and sound."[34]

Renan objected to Becker's theory because he alleged that it implied "the necessary and almost material production of language." He insisted

---

[29] Ibid., p. 92.

[30] Ibid., p. 94.

[31] Karl Ferdinand Becker, *Organism der Sprache* (Frankfurt am Main: G. F. Kettembeil, 1841), pp. 1–2.

[32] Ibid., p. 2.

[33] Ibid., p. 6.

[34] Ibid., p. 12.

with such German critics of Becker as Karl Wilhelm Ludwig Heyse that language was, on the contrary, an expression of human liberty.[35] Heyse had insisted that language was "no purely natural function. . . . It is a free spiritual activity, which gradually emerges in the individual and is variously exercised by different men. It is throughout an evolving property [*ein Werdendes*], not given in a finished state with man's physical organization."[36] Language therefore belonged "to man's spiritual essence not to the material organism."[37] Heyse reiterated the close association—the virtual identity—of language and reason. It was this "rational mind" that separated man from animals; and, more especially, "man is distinguished from animals by language. The animal has no language, just as it has no rational mind."[38]

Even in the new scientific philology, therefore, language retained a special quasi-sacred character. It was an aspect, perhaps even the essence, of humanity's higher nature. It marked a boundary not only between the human and the animal, but also between body and mind. Even though philologists were prepared to use terms drawn from life science to elucidate the nature and development of languages, there was a marked refusal to allow a merely physiological account of speech: in its psychic aspect, language belonged "to the spiritual being, not to the physical organism of man."[39]

Language was, moreover, not merely a token of man's partial separation from the rest of creation; it was also an emblem of his dominion over nature. Johann Peter Süssmilch in 1766 claimed the faculty of language to be "the sole means to attain the use of reason [and] to maintain mastery [*Herrschaft*] over the world and over all other creatures."[40] Johann Gottfried von Herder shared this notion of the role of speech in shaping human destiny. A dumb man, he declared, was no more than an animal—a pathetic, isolated being. Man "must either be subject to or rule over all, with an intelligence of which no animal is capable. . . . Be nothing or the Monarch of Creation through understanding! Wreak havoc, or make yourself language."[41]

---

[35] Renan, *De l'origine*, p. 39.

[36] Karl Wilhelm Ludwig Heyse, *System der Sprachwissenschaft* (Berlin: Ferd. Dümmler, 1856), p. 46.

[37] Ibid., p. 50.

[38] Ibid., p. 25.

[39] Ibid., p. 50.

[40] Johann Peter Süssmilch, *Versuch eines Beweises, dass die erste Sprache ihren Ursprung nicht vom Menschen, sondern allein vom Schöpfer erhalten haben* (Berlin: Buchladen der Realschule, 1766), pp. iii–iv; see also pp. 103–104.

[41] [Johann Gottfried von] Herder, *Abhandlung über den Ursprung der Sprache* (Berlin: C. F. Voss, 1772), p. 157.

In the nineteenth century Julien Joseph Virey (1775–1846) expressed a similar view of man's relation to nature. "We are," he insisted, "the head or thinking part of the organic realms," established to act as a "supreme moderator," and whose task was to create equilibrium and order in nature.[42] Man's superiority was, in part, expressed in his upright posture. But it depended principally upon his intellectual attributes; it was, above all, "by means of articulate language that we can augment indefinitely the symbols of all our ideas, and enrich our intelligence." This ability was conspicuously absent in the animals under human dominion; man alone possessed "the immense advantage of attaching a sign to each idea, and thus being able to preserve it, to communicate it to his fellow, and to transmit it to posterity."[43]

Materializing the Word

From the seventeenth to the first half of the nineteenth century language was thus invested with immense cultural significance. It served as a boundary category which reinforced a number of crucial hierarchies. Man's endowment with language distinguished him from the animal. Language indicated the duality of human nature—appertaining to a superior, spiritual aspect. The body was accordingly stigmatized as "the lesser part" of the human constitution.[44] There was, moreover, a strong association between word and power: man's linguistic ability gave him a license to rule over that which he could name.[45] Command of language was thus an active, masculine, mental attribute which facilitated the domination of a passive, material, feminine nature.[46]

The 1825 paper in which Jean-Baptiste Bouillaud made his first pronouncement on the relations of language and the brain was, according to the title, intended "to confirm the opinion of M. Gall on the seat of articulate language."[47] In the fourth volume of his *Anatomie et physiologie du système nerveux* (1818–19) Gall had sought to incorporate the faculty of language within his "organology": a system that maintained each major mental capacity must possess its own site within the brain. On the basis of

---

[42] J. J. Virey, *Histoire naturelle du genre humain*, 2nd ed., 4 vols. (Brussels: Aug. Wahlen, 1826), vol. 1, pp. 3, 10.

[43] Ibid., pp. 74–75, 76.

[44] Ibid., p. 78.

[45] V. N. Voloshinov, *Marxism and the Philosophy of Language* (New York: Seminar Press, 1973), pp. 74–75.

[46] Ludmilla Jordanova, *Sexual Visions: Images of Gender and Medicine between the Eighteenth and Twentieth Centuries* (New York: Harvester Press, 1989), pp. 19–42.

[47] Bouillaud, "Recherches cliniques," p. 25.

physiognomic observation Gall located the faculty of language above the orbital plate. He regarded this organ as the material basis of speech and other linguistic capabilities, and speculated that it explained the immutable laws of "general grammar" common to all nations.[48]

Besides physiognomy Gall also made use of comparative observations when seeking to identify the seats of the various mental powers. "Language," he maintained,

> is natural to animals; it is inherent in their being; it is the same for all the members of the same species; . . . all are fluent and all comprehend it perfectly. The attentive observer will easily be convinced that this language is much more developed than is usually supposed above all in the most intelligent species.

Not only could animals comprehend their own language: they were even capable of understanding "the arbitrarily formed languages of man."[49] Anatomy confirmed these behavioral observations. In birds the "greater the cerebral mass placed above the internal part of the bulb, the greater a species' aptitude for language."[50] Gall felt authorized to conclude that "speech . . . is an effect, a creation of our internal faculties; and . . . that a particular organ of the brain presides over this admirable function."[51]

He thus both identified the faculty of language with a determinate bodily structure and extended this power to animals. Thereby he simultaneously violated two of the boundaries that the traditional concept of language guarded. Gall was clearly also widening the scope of what counted as language in an unsettling way by including various forms of animal communication under that rubric.

Despite its stated aim, Bouillaud's paper is equivocal on these issues. At times it seems to uphold the sacred notion of language that Gall's text had challenged. Thus Bouillaud asserted that "man is the only animal who truly enjoys, in its full extent, the noble privilege of speech: . . . (and certainly it is not one of his lesser prerogatives)." Elsewhere he underlined the point by describing language as "the great faculty by which man is distinguished among all the animals."[52]

Bouillaud thus seemed to endorse the special character of language as a quality that raised humanity above the natural world. But even here this

---

[48] Franz-Joseph Gall, *Anatomie et physiologie du système nerveux en générale, et du cerveau en particulier, avec des observations sur la possibilité de reconnaître plusiers dispositions intellectuelles et morales de l'homme et des animaux, par la configuration du leurs têtes*, 4 vols. (Paris: N. Maze, 1818–19), vol. 4, p. 58.

[49] Ibid., pp. 63–64.

[50] Ibid., p. 65.

[51] Ibid., p. 68.

[52] Ibid., pp. 30, 43.

superiority is somewhat compromised by the insertion into both these passages of the presumption that man *is* an animal, even if uniquely endowed. Moreover, Bouillaud's assertion that man alone enjoyed language in its *full* extent was also double-edged: it implied that humanity's linguistic distinction was relative rather than absolute. Other animals might also possess some, if only limited, capacity for language.

When he came to explain the grounds for the distinction between man and "other" animals, the extent of Bouillaud's departure from established views of the nature of language became evident:

> if someone asks . . . why animals do not speak, we do not reply along with certain naturalists, that it is merely because they lack suitably arranged external organs for the articulation of sounds, but we add that these animals are deprived of speech because nature has denied them the internal organ, the cerebral centre that coordinates the movements by means of which man expresses, through the medium of words, the operations of his mind [*entendement*].[53]

This passage is at once disingenuous and boldly subversive. Previous "naturalists" had not, in fact, maintained that animals were incapable of speech because of the configuration of their vocal organs. On the contrary, the standard position was that there were no physical grounds why certain animals should not speak as well as man. Some animals, such as parrots, were, as Descartes had noted, able to articulate words. What they lacked was not the corporeal organization requisite for speech, but the intellectual capacity to employ words in a meaningful manner. Even when organic characters were invoked to explain an animal's inabilty to speak these structural peculiarities were related to the intellectual discrepancy between man and beast. Virey, for example, held that "the orangutang could, it is true, articulate sounds almost like a man . . . ; but nature, with truly extraordinary foresight, did not wish that an animal should join in human conversation, and that the idiocies of the beast could be mingled with the reasoning of rational beings." The orangutang's larynx accordingly possessed a special conformation to make speech impossible.[54]

What Bouillaud now implied was that animal inarticulacy did indeed have an organic basis; they lacked the cerebral organization necessary for speech. But the converse of this proposition was far more significant. Man spoke because he *did* possess an "internal organ" for the articulation of words located in the frontal lobes of the brain. Pathology proved that "these lobes truly are the prime mover, the mainspring [*ressort*], and so to speak the soul [*ame*] of the vital instruments for the articulation of sounds."[55]

---

[53] Ibid., p. 41.
[54] Virey, *Histoire naturelle*, p. 75.
[55] Bouillaud, "Recherches cliniques," p. 40.

Previous authors might have agreed upon the need for a "soul" to put the organs of speech into motion. But they would have recoiled from the notion so blithely expressed by Bouillaud that this soul might itself be a material entity. His invocation of the soul also sits uneasily with the mechanistic imagery that permeates this sentence. This assertion that the cerebral lobes might be the soul of speech tends to negate the earlier passage where Bouillaud writes in conventional terms of language as the means whereby "man . . . communicates his thoughts, expresses his feelings, and so to speak paints the movements of his soul."[56]

Bouillaud apparently mitigated the force of his embodiment of the moving force of language by insisting that speech was a complex phenomenon, and that he was concerned only with one part of it. The act of speaking comprised, he claimed, two distinct phenomena: "the faculty of creating words and symbols of our ideas, of retaining a memory of them, and that of articulating the same words. There is so to speak an interior speech and an exterior speech: the latter is no more than the expression of the former." Bouillaud's discourse was concerned only with the external, motor aspect of speech, not with its internal, intellectual side. His localization of the organ that presided over the movements of speaking might therefore seem to leave untouched the "higher" psychic and intellectual linguistic phenomena. But he went on to assert that there was in principle no reason why these phenomena should not be assigned a material basis. By making the distinction between internal and external aspects of speech all he was asserting was that "The nervous organization [*système nerveux*] that presides over the formation of signs is not the same as the one that produces the movements of the organs of speech."[57]

In subsequent presentations of his thesis Bouillaud emphasized that while Gall had been preoccupied with the intellectual side of the faculty of language, he was more concerned with its "mechanical element."[58] This bias had the additional effect of serving to emphasize the mundane and corporeal aspects of the phenomena. Language, from this viewpoint was but one form of muscular contraction innervated by a determinate region of the brain; it was not fundamentally different from any other of the voluntary bodily motions. In materializing the principle of articulate language Bouillaud also almost incidentally rendered the "higher" intellectual function of volition incarnate.

The operations that Bouillaud performed upon human speech can be usefully compared to Marx and Engels' discussion of language in *The Ger-*

[56] Ibid., p. 29.
[57] Ibid., p. 43.
[58] J.-B. Bouillaud, "Exposition de nouveaux faits à l'appui de l'opinion qui localise dans les lobules antérieures du cerveau le principe législateur de la parole; examen préliminaire des objections dont cette opinion a été le sujet," *Bullétin de l'Académie Royale de Médecine* 4 (1839–40): 282–328, p. 283.

man Ideology. This text sets out quite explicitly to undermine the mystified concept of language propounded by "philosophers." This notion was deemed inseparable from the reified notions of mind favored by the bourgeoisie. "Spirit," in Marx and Engels' view, "is afflicted with the curse of being 'burdened' with matter, which here makes its appearance in the form of agitated layers of air, sounds, in short, of language."[59] Just as philosophers had tried to give thought an independent existence, so they had tried to detach language from the material and social conditions of its existence.[60]

Bouillaud lacked any notion of language as something emerging from and dependent upon social intercourse—upon what Marx and Engels called "life." But he did in his own way bring language down to earth. More particularly, he brought it into the brain insisting that this was the true site of the faculty philosophers had insisted belonged to humanity's spiritual aspect. Thereby he also took a significant step towards embodying the metaphysicians' "mind." Bouillaud himself claimed as much at the end of an account of some experimental researches on the functions of the brain—in the course of which he had systematically violated the supposed categorical boundaries between man and animal. The "frontal region of the brain," he maintained, "is the seat of several intellectual faculties." This was he considered "the place to recall the facts we have published to prove that in man it is in the anterior part of the brain that resides the principle of the faculty of speech, of creating the representative signs of ideas and feelings; [a] faculty which constitutes one of the most sublime appanages of our species."[61] On Bouillaud's premises, the "sublimity" of language had, however, to reconcile itself with the mundaneness of its anatomical domicile.

The Grotesque Symposium

The second moment in the unfolding of the nineteenth-century discourse on language and the brain occurred in Paris under the Second Empire. An understanding of the political context is relevant to a reading of this episode. This was a period in which the overt expression of political views was rigidly controlled: the government of Napoleon III had "refined re-

---

[59] Karl Marx and Frederick Engels, *The German Ideology* (Moscow: Progress Publishers, 1964), p. 41.

[60] Ibid., p. 491.

[61] J.-B. Bouillaud, "Recherches expérimentales sur les fonctions du cerveau (lobes cérébraux) en général, et sur celles de sa portion antérieure en particulier," *Journal de Physiologie expérimentale et pathologique* 10 (1830): 36–98, pp. 97–98.

pression into an art."[62] As a result, it was also a period of what Edward Timms writing of nineteenth-century Vienna has called an "ideological saturation" of the culture—a state of affairs that endowed a wide range of symbolic interactions with a political import.[63] Opposition to the regime retreated into traditional cultural rituals such as the carnival; even these performances were, however, subject to scrutiny.[64] Under such conditions, new occasions and forms of interaction were found for the necessarily coded expression of political sentiment.[65]

Paul Broca was typical of those of liberal and republican sympathies who were obliged to live and work under these conditions. As Francis Schiller remarks, if Broca had given public vent to his privately stated opinions during the first dozen years of the Second Empire, "he would have had to sacrifice all else."[66] His utterances and actions were accordingly confined to professional and scientific activity in such fields as physical anthropology and anatomy as well as clinical medicine. Such activity did not, however, represent a complete withdrawal from the political; rather it constituted a pragmatic acceptance of the conditions under which a political agenda could with safety be pursued.

Because the obvious opportunities for political expression were precluded, other less well-policed public spaces were adapted or created for this purpose. Broca was, in particular, the leading figure in the foundation in 1859 of the Société d'Anthropologie de Paris, a forum in which a range of overtly scientific, and therefore safe, but also highly charged issues could be debated with little interference.[67]

Scientific controversy could serve as a proxy for or adjunct to political debate because of the extensive and pervasive character of factional discourse in nineteenth-century France. The ideologies of the period were

[62] Gay, *Cultivation of Hatred*, p. 248.

[63] Edward Timms, *Karl Kraus Apocalyptic Satirist: Culture and Catastrophe in Habsburg Vienna* (New Haven: Yale University Press, 1986), pp. 28, 124–128.

[64] Robert J. Bezucha, "Masks of Revolution: A Study of Popular Culture during the Second French Republic," in Roger Price (ed.), *Revolution and Reaction: 1848 and the Second French Republic* (London: Croom Helm, 1975), pp. 236–253.

[65] See: Peter McPhee, *A Social History of France, 1780–1880* (London: Routledge, 1992), p. 187.

[66] Francis Schiller, *Paul Broca: Founder of French Anthropology, Explorer of the Brain* (Berkeley: University of California Press, 1969), p. 279.

[67] Joy Harvey, "Evolutionism Transformed: Positivists and Materialists in the *Société d'Anthropologie de Paris* from Second Empire to Third Republic," in David Oldroyd (ed.), *The Wider Domain of Evolutionary Thought* (London: Reidel, 1983), pp. 289–310; M. Hammond, "Anthropology as a Weapon of Social Combat in late-Nineteenth-Century France," *Journal of the History of the Behavioural Sciences* 16 (1980): 118–32. For a more general discussion of the agenda of the Société see: Elizabeth A. Williams, "The Science of Man: Anthropological Thought and Institutions in Nineteenth-Century France," Indiana University PhD, 1983, chapter 3.

so extensive as to constitute veritable worldviews: there was, in Claude Nicolet's words, "a republican 'science' . . . in the pedagogic sense of the term. There was a republican *philosophy.* . . . There was above all a republican *morality*."[68] Nicolet notes that this republican cosmology was sustained and developed in the course of the nineteenth century in opposition to rival systems. Perhaps the most important of these conflicts was that with the Catholic-royalist reaction to the political and cultural consequences of the Revolution.

"Liberty" was the key value of the republican moral order; indeed, in the political iconography of the period Liberty and the Republic were often identified.[69] Of all the trammels upon freedom of thought and of expression none was more abhorrent to republicans than those associated with the power and authority of the Catholic church. The close alliance between church and state during the Second Empire strengthened the impression that these were merely different sides of the same system of repression.

The republican emphasis on liberty contributed to what Zeldin describes as the movement's tendency to approximate to a form of "permanent revolution."[70] Republicanism was, in other words, characterized by a tendency to question and challenge authority of all kinds. At the same time, however, as they sought to contest and subvert existing systems and hierachies, and particularly those connected with the theocratic notions of their political enemies, republicans were also engaged in a more constructive endeavor. Throughout the nineteenth century they sought to achieve an account of human nature free from all theological concepts: to attain, in short, "a desacralization and a naturalization of thought."[71]

The debates in the Société d'Anthropologie partook of both these aspects of the republican ethic. There was on the one hand a fearless questioning of accepted authority—a refusal to accept that anything was sacred. While, on the other hand, in the course of these debates the

---

[68] Claude Nicolet, *L'idée républicaine en France (1789–1924): Essai d'histoire critique* (Paris: Gallimard, 1982), p. 11. This conflict between what were effectively rival worldviews can be traced back to the attack upon the cosmological foundations of the old regime that occurred during the French Revolution; for an illuminating discussion see: Lynn Hunt, *Politics, Culture, and Class in the French Revolution* (Berkeley: University of California Press, 1984), pp. 87–88.

[69] Maurice Agulhon, *Marianne into Battle: Republican Imagery and Symbolism in France, 1789–1880* (Cambridge: Cambridge University Press, 1981), pp. 38–39, 82.

[70] Theodore Zeldin, *France 1848–1945: Politics and Anger* (Oxford: Oxford University Press, 1979), p. 130.

[71] Nicolet, *L'idée républicaine*, p. 11.

lineaments of an alternative hierarchy based on a fully naturalistic account of human nature became visible. It was during one such debate that Broca's "contribution" to the history of aphasiology was first advanced.

The discussion of language arose as a modulation of a prior debate on the question of the "Big Heads." At issue was the possibility of discerning a direct correlation between cranial or brain size and intelligence. In the course of the argument a variety of "proofs" were presented in support of or to discredit the proposition. These included such equivocal and faintly comic objects as a skull that may or may not have been that of Descartes, and a hat which had indubitably belonged to Georges Cuvier.

A strong faction within the Society insisted that such a correlation was evident. On 21 February 1861, for instance, Broca declared that:

> It is therefore infinitely probable that, of all the men whose brains have so far been weighed, Cuvier and Lord Byron, two great men, two men of genius, who number among the outstanding figures of our age, are the ones who have possessed most cerebral mass. It appears to me impossible to attribute this result to pure coincidence and not to admit that these two men owed the supremacy of their intelligence to the volume of their brain.[72]

There was, in other words, a need to admit that there was "a well-defined relationship between the mass of the brain and the power of the intelligence."[73]

This was a point to insist on because, if conceded, it ruptured a crucial boundary between spirit and matter, mind and body. If the "power of the intelligence" varied with the size of the brain, then mind was not independent of and superior to the corporeal part of man. The very crudity of the language by which this claim was expressed emphasized the effect of this strategy of materialization: at one point, for instance, Broca spoke of the possibility of "weighing minds"[74]—a paradoxical coupling of terms normally deemed to belong to utterly different realms. Intelligence—a "spiritual" quality—was on these premises dependent on the amount of cerebral stuff an individual carried within his skull.

Not all members of the Society were prepared to allow the legitimacy of this maneuver. Broca's principal antagonist in the affair of the Big Heads was Pierre Gratiolet (1815–65), a leading neuroanatomist. Gratiolet maintained that the possession of a small brain did not necessarily imply that an individual was endowed with a "vulgar spirit." The dimen-

---

[72] *Bulletins de la Société d'Anthropologie de Paris* 2 (1861): 77.
[73] Ibid., p. 154.
[74] Ibid., p. 160.

sions of Cuvier's hat—as opposed to the weight of his brain—were not, in the light of Gratiolet's inquiries in the millinery trade, exceptional.[75] The irony of the fact that savants should rely upon the testimony of hatters to settle so important a question went unremarked.[76]

Gratiolet also demurred at the crassness of both the language his opponents had used in their contributions to this debate and of their anatomical techniques. He argued that by simply ripping the brain from the skull they ignored important relations of the organ that needed to be studied *in situ*: "One wants only to see the brain. One takes this king away from his empire, one weighs it in isolation, one wishes, were it possible, to weigh only the cortical layers!" In place of this crude and irreverent *levelling* attitude to the brain, Gratiolet advocated a more qualitative approach to deciding the relative "dignity" of different parts of the nervous system. He insisted that an aesthetic appreciation which took account of the form and degree of perfection of the brain was of at least as much relevance as a merely quantitiative approach. For Gratiolet the human brain was a thing of beauty as well as of mass.[77] It was, moreover, an analogue of the embodiment of political authority in the traditional polity.

In contrast to the homogenizing tendency of the weighers, Gratiolet represented a more aristocratic sensibility, as evinced by his disdain for "vulgar" spirits. His was a differentiated, hierarchical vision of the brain. It was also an organicist rather than mechanistic vision. For Gratiolet, "the frontal lobes are, so to speak, the flower of the brain, and everything, in effect, indicates that they possess a superior physiological dignity." Far from being crude matter, the structure of the brain evinced an underlying plan or idea so that: "above weight we place the form, but above the form we put the vital energy, the intrinsic power of the brain."[78] Intelligence depended not upon the weight of the brain but upon the complete achievement of the design executed by this immaterial energy.

Gratiolet thus insisted upon the categorical distinctions that Broca had sought to undermine. During the session of 18 April he supplied the theological context for his earlier contributions. "I believe," he avowed, "in the existence of the soul"; and this was for Gratiolet an entity beyond the

[75] Ibid., pp. 428–30.

[76] As Steven Shapin has pointed out, however, it was a well-established practice for natural philosophers to credit "vulgar" testimony provided the subject matter lay within the area of expertise of a witness: *A Social History of Truth: Civility and Science in Seventeenth-Century England* (Chicago: University of Chicago Press, 1994), pp. 218–19. In this instance, the tradesmen in question were clearly competent—indeed, uniquely well placed—to offer an opinion on prevalent hat sizes.

[77] *Bulletins*, pp. 252–253.

[78] Ibid., p. 258.

reach of the tools of physical science.[79] He did not, however, maintain that medical science was irrelevant to the determination of psychological questions: according to his biographer, "the conclusion of Gratiolet's profound meditations, of his patient investigations, of his delicate dissections" had been that "thought, spirit, or the soul . . . is an essence, being *par excellence*, and not at all a mere phenomenon."[80] He expounded a spiritualist philosophy which, while scientifically informed, was fully compatible with a Christian and hierarchical conception of the natural order. The brain was "king" and the body its "empire."[81]

Gratiolet's understanding of language was correspondingly conservative and orthodox. A text of 1857 repeated the venerable identification of language with reason: "in effect," Gratiolet maintained, "human thought is an internal language; it is therefore very difficult to formulate an idea of intelligence independent of this superior faculty."[82] Gratiolet distinguished different kinds of language. The "automatic and spontaneous language of cries and gestures," for instance, was common to both man and animals. But "algebraic" or symbolic language was "altogether the work of the spirit" and therefore exclusive to humans.[83] The rigid distinction between human and animal modes of communication which Gall had blurred was thus reinstated.

This was indeed the chief basis of the distinction between man and beast; it was "absolutely false to say . . . that man differs from animals only by degree [*du plus ou moins*]."[84] Even in microencephalic monsters human reason retained its specific character. Such beings were able to speak intelligently whereas a monkey which possessed far more cerebral substance was dumb. Gratiolet accordingly proposed that the taxonomic space occupied by the human species should be designated the "*kingdom of the word*."[85]

While language served to segregate the human from the animal, it also created no less significant affinities with other realms. The faculty for

---

[79] Ibid., p. 270.

[80] Louis Grandeau, *Pierre Gratiolet: Sa vie et travaux* (Paris: J. Hetzel, 1865), p. 6.

[81] *Bulletins*, p. 252.

[82] François Leuret and Pierre Gratiolet, *Anatomie comparée du système nerveux considéré dans ses rapports avec l'intelligence, comprenant la description de l'encéphale et de la moelle rachidienne, des recherches sur le développement, le volume, le poids, la structure de ces organes chez l'homme et les animaux vertébrés; l'histoire du système ganglionaire des animaux articulés et des mollusques, et l'exposé de la relation qui existe entre la perfection progressive de ces centres nerveux et l'état des facultés instinctives, intellectuelles et morales*, 2 vols, (Paris: J.-B. Baillière, 1839–57), vol. 2, pp. 639–640.

[83] Ibid., pp. 664–665.

[84] Ibid., p. 671.

[85] Ibid., p. 687.

representation and symbolic expression allowed humans to participate "in the creative power of God. It is true that God alone creates substances, but he has communicated to man alone the power to create and to define forms." Because of this quasi-divine attribute, man was not only apart from but was above the rest of the creation: he was "king of living nature."[86]

Gratiolet reiterated this transcendent concept of language in the course of the 1861 debate at the Société d'Anthropologie. On 18 April he declared that:

> I need not say that, not dividing the brain at all according to the primary faculties of mind, I make no attempt to determine the seat of the faculty of language. In effect, thought and word are synonymous, and wherever there is a free thought, there is a language which radiates through all the mechanisms [*appareils*] of the body, like the light of the soul. Human speech is not only in the voice, it is wherever there is the possibility of movement: the mute speak with their fingers, the hand that traces signs speaks to the eyes; painting and sculpture have a language; the Word is the principle and the purpose of the human soul.[87]

Here language is identified with the "higher," intellectual and spiritual part of human nature. It suffuses and empowers the body without being dependent upon the flesh. Language resists, in particular, any attempt to tie it to some specific site within the body.

Gratiolet articulated this view in response to a starkly different notion of the nature of language and of its relation to the body that had emerged in the course of the Society's discussions. The issue of the Big Heads had at an early stage turned into a debate about the possibility of cerebral localization: about whether there was, in effect, a division of labour within the material substrate of mind.[88]

On 21 February Ernest Aubertin (who was Bouillaud's son-in-law) had made the point that:

> the brain [*encéphale*] . . . is a complex organ, with various and multiple functions, and it is therefore natural that the total volume of this organ does not give an exact measure of the development of the intelligence. But if, instead of considering the organ in its entirety one examines its various parts, one discovers more precise facts; one knows, for instance, that the most lofty cerebral functions have a relation to the development of the frontal lobes, and if

---

[86] Ibid., pp. 673, 662.

[87] *Bulletins*, p. 274.

[88] For a discussion of the ideological ramifications of this metaphor see: Roger J. Cooter, *The Cultural Meaning of Popular Science: Phrenology and the Organization of Consent in Nineteenth-Century Britain* (Cambridge: Cambridge University Press, 1985), pp. 111–112.

it is true that certain men of genius have had a brain that was not as a whole large, their busts and their portraits show us that at least the frontal part of this organ was well developed.[89]

This was a reiteration of the tenets of Gall's organology.

Gratiolet responded that the question of whether particular parts of the cerebrum had a special relation to individual mental faculties was undecided. Later, however, he expressed a stronger skepticism about the possibility of performing such localizations: "In a general manner," he declared, "I believe with M. Flourens that intelligence is one, that the cerebrum [*cerveau*] is one, that it acts above all as unitary organ." This did not, however, exclude the possibility that particular parts of the cerebrum might be specially dedicated to certain functions; but none was *exclusively* and uniquely devoted to some such task.[90]

Auburtin brushed aside such qualifications and concluded that Gratiolet had avowed himself an adherent of Pierre Flourens' holistic concept of cerebral function.[91] Such a conclusion might, he conceded, be tenable if "one has only studied cerebral physiology by means of vivisections"; anatomy and "pathological physiology" conduced, however, to a contrary opinion. Thus damage to the middle lobes of the brain produced quite different effects than injuries to the anterior part of the cerebrum. A lesion of the frontal lobes "does not impair either sensibility or motility; but it does abolish the faculty of language."[92]

Language thus entered the debate as an exemplary or paradigmatic case. In Auburtin's words, "it is enough to establish a single localization for the principle of localization to be established."[93] This operation would, moreover, serve the cause of grounding intelligence in matter. The fact that language of all the faculties of mind was chosen as the test case was, given the cultural values invested in this attribute, of particular strategic importance.

Gratiolet acknowledged this by addressing Bouillaud's and Auburtin's claims directly. He denied that there was any necessary or invariable relationship between damage to the anterior lobes and impairment of language. He argued, moreover, that the evidence of comparative anatomy was also incompatible with the claims of the localizers. Apes, he pointed out, "also possess anterior lobes, and these lobes are divided as in man"; the ape, however, "does not speak." Gratiolet maintained that if there was

[89] *Bulletins*, pp. 71–72.
[90] Ibid., pp. 74, 78.
[91] For Flourens' doctrines see: Edwin Clarke and L. S. Jacyna, *Nineteenth-Century Origins of Neuroscientific Concepts* (Berkeley: University of California Press, 1987), pp. 250–253.
[92] *Bulletins*, p. 79.
[93] Ibid., p. 213.

indeed a material organ of language then apes should at least possess some rudimentary linguistic capacity.[94] He accordingly felt justified to conclude that all the attempts at localization that have been put forward so far lack any foundation: "These are great efforts, to be sure, the efforts of Titans! But when one wishes to seize celestial truth from the top of these *Babels*, the edifice collapses."[95] Gratiolet's choice of Biblical allusion is telling. The story of the Tower of Babel showed the folly of human hubris; in this instance God punished men's efforts to reach forbidden heights by depriving them of the gift of a common language in which they had previously communicated.

On 21 March Broca made clear his own position in this controversy. Just as Gratiolet confessed his faith in the existence of the soul, so Broca affirmed his own credo: "I believe . . . in the principle of localizations." Earlier in the session he had argued that this was an idea which was peculiarly well attuned to the spirit of the age. While he was far from hostile to the aristocratic notion that progress was the work of a few "great men," Broca also stressed the milieu in which these individuals were obliged to operate and which to a great extent determined the success or failure of their ideas. "One can say," he maintained,

> that when a doctrine obtains a rapid success, it is because its author has the good fortune to promulgate it at an opportune time, because he has formulated and developed an idea which was of the tendency of the epoch, and which already existed under a still vague form in a large number of minds.[96]

This Comtean law of the historical development of ideas explained the success that Gall's central doctrine had enjoyed. The principle of cerebral localization was

> the natural consequence of the philosophic movement of the nineteenth century, for the time is past when one could say without hesitation, in the name of metaphysics, that, the soul being simple, the brain [*cerveau*]—anatomy notwithstanding—must also be simple. Everything concerning the relations of mind with matter has been put into question, and in the midst of the uncertainties that surround the solution of this great problem, anatomy and physiology, until now reduced to silence, must at last raise their voice.[97]

Anatomy and physiology thus spoke with the voice of modernity.

[94] Ibid., p. 268.
[95] Ibid., p. 269.
[96] Ibid., p. 190.
[97] Ibid., p. 191.

The "philosophic movement of the nineteenth century" was therefore one in which the old hierarchical relation between spirit and matter was contested and inverted; where the authority of metaphysics over physical science was challenged; where previously suppressed voices would at last be heard. The paradox was that these voices were now only to be heard by virtue of the silence of others; and it was this silence that was the subject of the new discourse.

As Auburtin remarked it had to be so. Whatever advantage Gratiolet might discern in experimental as opposed to clinical truth, in the case of language the question of localization could only be determined by a study of the effects of human injury and disease—"since animals do not speak." It was true that Bouillaud had shown that dogs deprived of their frontal lobes ceased to bark; but, "barking cannot be compared to human language."[98]

There was, however, an ambivalence at work in this concurrent erection of distinctions and drawing of analogies. Although barking dogs were not speaking humans, the fact that they ceased to bark when their frontal lobes were ablated was a matter of some significance and comfort for those concerned to discover a cerebral basis for language. Moreover, although the clinic rather than the laboratory was obviously the site in which to explore these questions, the two locales were not necessarily exclusive; it was possible to transfer the language and procedures of the one to the other.

Thus of the case histories Auburtin adduced to support his claims, one conformed to the conventions of the classic clinical description. A woman aged fifty-five years fell down some steps injuring her head. Eventually, she lost the power of speech while retaining her intelligence and the power to move her tongue and lips. An autopsy revealed extensive abcesses in both frontal lobes.[99]

But the other history transgressed the limitations of these conventions. This was the case of a soldier who had shot himself through the forehead thus exposing without injuring the frontal lobes. He survived in this state for several hours with both intelligence and speech unimpaired. While in this state, Auburtin reported,

> the following experiment [*expérience*] was performed on him. While someone questioned him, the blade of a spatula was applied to the frontal lobes; pressure was gradually increased, and speech was suddenly suspended; the word he had started [to enunciate] was cut in two. The faculty of language returned when the compression ceased.[100]

[98] Ibid., p. 217.
[99] Ibid., p. 216.
[100] Ibid., pp. 217–218.

Here the dichotomies of the clinical and the experimental collapsed. The doctor was in this instance able actively to intervene rather than rest content with the passive observation of the "experiments" that nature had performed on the human body. He had, in effect, become nature's laboratory assistant. The ontological status of the patient/subject is also equivocal; he is effectively reduced to the status of an experimental animal serving the interests of science as long as he survives. It was, Auburtin maintained, only this opportunity to apply precise pressure to the frontal region that obviated various objections that had been made to other attempts to corroborate the localization of language in that part of the brain.

Two weeks later Broca presented a case of his own designed to make the same point. This was the story of "Tan," which has attained the status of a classic—perhaps even *the* classic—in the canon of aphasiology.[101] He did in fact do more than present the case: the exemplary brain was itself produced as additional ocular evidence for the localizationist claim that the word was subject to the natural shocks that flesh is heir to. The brain was to be preserved in the Musée Dupuytren as a trophy to the scientific conquest of the definitive faculty of the human mind.

Conclusion

It is difficult to discern any clear-cut winner in the debate at the Société d'Anthropologie. This was in part because rather than engaging in a genuine dialogue the participants tended to talk past each other while enunciating and elaborating their own position. As Gratiolet remarked late in the process, "it is often the case that instead of achieving understanding through discussion one increases the distance."[102] This could, no doubt, be seen as another legacy of the Tower of Babel: even men of science lacked a common tongue.

There was nonetheless a clear movement within the text of the debate towards a demystified view of language as a bodily action rather than as a quasi-divine attribute. Language was assimilated to the model of organic function. Speech might be a "higher" function in the sense that it was, as Auburtin readily conceded,[103] an exceptionally complex bodily operation;

---

[101] Paul Broca, "Remarques sur le siège de la faculté du langage articulé, suivies d'une observation d'aphémie (perte de la parole)," *Bulletins de la Société Anatomique de Paris* 6 (1861): 326–57. The patient's name was Leborgne; however, he became known as "Tan" after the only syllable he was able to enunciate. For an account of the case see: Schiller, *Paul Broca*, pp. 181–86.

[102] *Bulletins*, p. 422.

[103] Ibid., p. 214.

but there was no reason why it should be considered as in principle different from digestion or indeed any other form of muscular movement.[104]

In his contribution to the debate Hippolyte-Félicité-Paul de Jouvencel
presented this achievement as a new stage in a process of gradual intellectual mastery over the secrets of the body. He reminded the members of
the Society that: "We here are . . . a learned body [*société savante*]; our
aim is to constitute a science of man." For all his undoubted credentials
as a man of science, Gratiolet's recent contribution to this endeavour
was flawed because he had allowed "metaphysics" to pollute the purity
of his discourse. Metaphysics might have its place; but it had no use in
understanding man conceived as "a distinct, observable and measurable
object."[105]

The new positive science of man must encompass all aspects of its subject. The ancients had understood digestion no better than they did
thought; the mysteries of the former function had now succumbed to
science. Jouvencel recognized, however, that special barriers protected
mind from the intrusion of the scientific gaze. He embodied these in the
person of a "Metaphysics" who confronted the searcher after truth and
announced:

> Stop! you [*tu*] can go no further. I shall establish for you the sole certainty
> that you can attain on this subject, I shall attest that you can know no more.
> Be consoled, the possession of an immortal soul which makes you equal to a
> god, the faculty of language which is the justification of your majesty and
> liberty, do these not suffice for your glory![106]

The answer was, of course, that such consolations were not a sufficient
compensation for ignorance: there could be no inviolable areas from
which science was excluded.

Knowledge was, moreover, intimately related to power. We have,
Jouvencel boasted, "subdued the general forces of nature: we have made
electricity a messenger, light a sketch-artist [*dessinateur*], affinity an industrial worker." If for Gratiolet man was the "king" of the natural world, for
Jouvencel enlightened humanity was nature's taskmaster. Why, he asked,
should science not proceed to gain equal mastery over the forces "by

---

[104] The question of whether aphemia signified a lesion of the "higher" intellectual faculties
or was merely a motor disorder was one which exercised Broca: "Remarques," pp. 333–37.

[105] *Bulletins*, p. 284. Such appropriation of the epithet of "science" and "scientific" was
highly tendentious. The spiritualist philosophy at which Jouvencal's polemic was largely directed claimed that its own method was scientific. See: John I. Brooks, *The Eclectic Legacy:
Academic Philosophy and the Human Sciences in Nineteenth-Century France* (Newark: University of Delaware Press, 1998), esp. p. 44.

[106] Ibid., p. 288.

which we ourselves operate?" If some "business profit" was attached to this kind of knowledge, the process of discovery would be accelerated.[107] From a late twentieth-century perspective, when the life sciences are indeed pursued with an eye to profit, and when the knowledge so gleaned offers the means to engineer new bodies, this passage has a peculiar resonance.

The insistence on the need to press ahead with the project of seeking a naturalistic account of mental faculties—and of language in particular—could thus be presented rhetorically as an assertion of intellectual freedom and as part of a wider pattern of progress. In a context where state and church were in league to preserve authority and tradition, such a call for unhindered inquiry, even when it touched on aspects of human nature that had previously been classed as sacred, possessed a subversive political significance. Jouvencel's assimilation of thought to the "lowly" bodily function of digestion, as well as his insinuation that there was a "mechanism" of mind to be discovered, should also be read in this context.[108] Such maneuvers may be viewed as part of a strategy of demystification of the sacred icons elevated by the established powers. In this sense, it is possible to speak of the 1861 debate at the Société d'Anthropologie as carnivalesque in some of its aspects. The embodiment of language was one instance of the secular process of desanctification whereby, in Marx's words, "all that is holy is profaned."[109]

Reviewing the trend toward naturalism in nineteenth-century culture, however, a contemporary lamented what he called "the tendency to self-debasement . . . in the shape of a scientific speculation, the scope of which is to veil all man's higher affinities and instincts, and to throw into strong relief his affinities with the creatures below him."[110] This author was determined to insist on the sacred character of human language. What from one perspective appeared a triumph of reason and science was from another an abomination.

It is important, however, to recognize that a reading of the text of the 1861 debate solely in terms of radical reversal would be misleading because partial. In his discussion of the place of politics in nineteenth-century French life, Theodore Zeldin remarks that: "The radicals who tried so hard to destroy Catholic teaching and introduce a lay morality never quite caught up with the fact that the morality they preached was very

---

[107] Ibid., p. 286.

[108] Ibid., p. 289.

[109] Quoted in Marshall Berman, *All That is Solid Melts Into Air* (New York: Penguin, 1988), p. 115.

[110] Edward Meyrick Goulburn, "Preface," to Frederick Bateman, *Darwinism Tested by Language* (London: Rivingtons, 1877), pp. xx–xxi.

little different from that of the Catholics."[111] Similarly, for all the evident rebellion implicit in the claims of the materializing tendency within the Société d'Anthropologie they shared a considerable body of values and assumptions with their apparent antagonists. The logocentricity of Western culture was, for example, preserved in Broca's notion of the foundations of social inequality: he quoted without demur Parchappe's assertion that a "talent for speaking or writing" raised certain individuals above the mediocre.[112]

More generally, the social vision that Broca offered in the course of his contributions to the debate was inscribed with a number of conventional assumptions about the differences between members of the species encompassed by the new "Science of Man," the constitution of which was the avowed aim of the Society. "Man," it transpired, encompassed a congeries of unequal beings. Broca took as unquestioned the view that professionals were more "intelligent" than manual workers;[113] that whites were inherently intellectually superior to other races; and that women's minds were inferior to men's.[114] It was left to Gratiolet to express mild reservations about this last generalization.[115] "Intelligence" remained an entirely unanalyzed category; its meaning was supposedly self evident.

In short, while the operations at work in the text of the debate may well have been directed towards the subversion of a particular ordering of persons and powers based on theocratic and spiritualist premises, profound hierarchical assumptions remained unchallenged. At most, the need for a supernatural underpinning of the inequalities of nineteenth-century bourgeois society was contested, but only in order to instate a naturalistic understanding of why such inequality was necessary and therefore just.[116]

---

[111] Zeldin, *France*, p. 22.

[112] *Bulletins*, p. 173. In a later debate Broca also displayed a yearning to retain language's special status as a signifier of man's special and superior status within the animal creation. See: Harrington, *Medicine*, pp. 50–51.

[113] Frederic Bateman in 1869 reported that: "With the view of verifying the accuracy of this statement [that the development of the higher faculties of the intellect varies in relation to the development of the anterior region of the skull], M. Broca examined the heads of thirty-two house-surgeons who had successively resided at Bicêtre during the years 1861–1862, and compared their dimensions with those of the heads of twenty-four porters attached to the various wards of the same hospital. This comparison resulted in the confirmation of the generally received opinion, that the anterior lobes are the seat of the highest order of intellectual faculties." "Aphasia or Loss of Speech in Cerebral Disease," *Journal of Mental Science* 15 (1870): 388fn.

[114] *Bulletins*, pp. 166, 172, 174, 176.

[115] Ibid., p. 244.

[116] It has been argued that all "carnivalesque" events serve to reinforce the hierarchies they apparently subvert. On this point see: Janet Beizer, *Ventriloquizing Bodies: Narratives of Hysteria in Nineteenth-Century France* (Ithaca: Cornell University Press, 1994), p. 217.

The brain in its diverse and yet regular forms and attributes now became the foundation of a natural order presided over by white males of the professional classes.[117] The brain-centered body in which the faculties of intelligence and dominion inhered was an elitist, masculine, classical formation, far removed from the bodily grotesque of popular culture. There were parts of the text that the spirit of carnival never reached.

[117] The establishment of an organ of language in the brain can also be viewed as a crucial moment in the process of the very constitution of "man" as an entity within whose body the physiological and anatomical conditions of knowledge were inscribed. See the remarks in: Michel Foucault, *The Order of Things: An Archaeology of the Human Sciences* (London: Tavistock, 1970), p. 319.

THREE

THE DISCOURSE OF APHASIA

*The essential and invaluable element in every morality is that it
is a protracted constraint.*
(Friedrich Nietzsche, Beyond Good and Evil, *Section 188)*

PAUL BROCA's contribution to the 1861 debate at the Société
d'Anthropologie, together with a number of later cases he published in which speech loss was accompanied by apparently determinate cerebral lesions, marked an epoch in the debate on the relations of
language and the brain. Broca's claims were not uncontroversial; on the
contrary his identification of the third frontal convolution of the left (or,
at least, the dominant) hemisphere as the "seat" of the faculty of language
was hotly debated. But the argument had taken on a novel register. By the
mid-1860s it was no longer a question of *whether* language was, in some
sense, represented in the brain. The issue had become that of *how* this
representation was to be conceptualized.

A few diehard opponents of the very idea of localization did remain,
but they became increasingly marginal and indeed irrelevant to the tendency of medical discourse. In 1865 Louis Francisque Lélut (1804–77)
took the opportunity of a discussion in the Académie de Médecine to
reaffirm that, while he was open to suasion on some issues, on certain
matters he remained inseparably wedded to views derived from "thirty or
forty years of study." Above all, Lélut refused to modify his attitude either
to the general attempt to "establish a relation between some fact or some
faculty of the mind, and some part of the central nervous system"; or to
the more particular endeavor to attribute "some part or the other of this
system to the faculty of language and to speech." All such efforts were "no
more or less than phrenology"—a "pseudo-science" which Lélut felt he
had already done quite enough to refute.[1]

He nonetheless condescended to address the more particular thesis that
the seat [*siège*] of language lay in the left hemisphere of the brain. He
found this proposition improbable on a priori grounds, and advanced a
number of "facts" designed to make it appear still less plausible. Thus Lélut

---

[1] "Discussion sur la faculté du langage articulé," *Bulletin de l'Académie Impériale de Médecine* 30 (1864–65): 173. Louis Francisque Lélut, *Qu'est-ce que la phrénologie? Ou essai sur
la significance et la valeur des systèmes de psychologie en général, et de celui de Gall en particulier*

cited the case of an epileptic the left side of whose brain was discovered at autopsy reduced to mush; this individual had, however, retained the power of speech to the end. Another fact took the form of a picture—"at this moment in my collection of sketches executed by myself at first hand [*sous les yeux*]"—of a carcinomatous cerebellum. In this case, speech had been impaired. Given such facts, Lélut saw no reason to deviate from his previous position on the question of the supposed localization of the faculty of language. He ended with a pun: "*mon siège est fait.*"[2]

This conceit was to prove ill advised. Lélut's challenge was immediately answered by the patriarch of the localizationist tribe, Jean-Baptiste Bouillaud, who adopted and elaborated upon his antagonist's play on words. Lélut had, Bouillaud declared, sought to lay *siège* to the localizationist citadel; the weapons with which he presumed to demolish this edifice were, however, pitifully inadequate. Bouillaud in effect subjected Lélut's contribution to a close textual criticism designed to show that, according to the canon of scientific discourse, his dialectical artillery was only competent to make ineffectual, if resounding, noise.

Bouillaud first remarked upon the brevity of Lélut's text: it occupied a mere two pages in the *Bullétin* of the Académie. Such terseness devalued the value of Lélut's contribution, making it seem slight and even frivolous. Such *laconisme* was, Bouillaud remarked, "unusual in this place."[3] A valid scientific presentation in an academy of medicine was therefore supposed to possess a certain gravity; weight, substance, and seriousness were all intertwined. Bouillaud's own text was in this regard exemplary. He developed his argument with tireless prolixity over several sessions of the Académie's meetings, filling seemingly endless pages of the published proceedings.[4]

Bouillaud also sought to problematize Lélut's appeal in his argument to certain matters of "fact." In so doing Bouillaud tacitly acknowledged the central, almost sacred, status of fact in scientific discourse. But he sought to show that Lélut's "facts" belonged in inverted commas; they were unworthy aspirants to this noble epithet. What Lélut called a "quite magnificent fact"—the story of the left hemisphere turned to mush without any impairment of speech—was for Bouillaud a conceptual monstrosity. It involved the notion of a cause with no effect. In terms of the organicist canon within which he operated the corollary of the dictum no

---

(Paris: Trinquart, 1836); idem, *Rejet de l'organologie de Gall, et de ses successeurs* (Paris: Fortin, Masson, 1843).

[2] Ibid., pp. 174–175.

[3] Ibid., p. 578.

[4] On the generation of the conventions defining valid forms of scientific prose see: Steven Shapin and Simon Schaffer, *Leviathan and the Air-Pump: Hobbes, Boyle, and the Experimental Life* (Princeton: Princeton University Press, 1985), pp. 62–65.

symptom without organic lesion was that a profound destruction of the brain *must* have functional consequences. "Facts" of the kind invoked by Lélut could lead only to:

> the *negation*, [to] the annihilation of all physiological and pathological science, and it is such a *fact* that M. Lélut . . . presents to us as *proof* that the seat of the faculty of speech does not lie in the anterior lobes of the brain.

This and Lélut's other instances were not genuine facts but "pseudo-facts," incompatible with the accepted rules of legitimate scientific language.[5]

As well as these matters of substance Bouillaud found fault with the style of his antagonist's performance. He had exercised his undoubted *vertu comique* in a genre where such jesting was vicious.[6] Lélut was thus rebuked for seeking to carnivalize the notion of localization, for trying to present it as an idea fit for laughter. This was merely an extension of the strategy that he had employed in his polemics against phrenology, parts of which, Bouillaud sternly remarked, "more resembled a comedy than a truly serious work."[7]

No one rose to defend Lélut from this onslaught. He himself seems to have been absent from the sessions at which Bouillaud spoke—or at least thought it prudent to maintain an "eloquent silence." By 1865 the notion that there was a cerebral basis for the faculty of language had achieved the status of an orthodoxy; there were few who would dispute its status as a scientific "fact." Those who would not recognize this were fit for scorn.

The claim was bolstered by its embedment in a wider localizationist concept of the structure and workings of the brain. Bouillaud stipulated the principal tenets of this system. The fundamental dogma of the new physiology of the brain was that this was a composite organ the various parts of which were dedicated to particular functions. There was, in effect, "a sort of cerebral *university*" compounded of the various mental faculties.[8] Secondly, it was possible to specify the "geography" or "topography" of these mental organs, to specify *where* in the brain a particular faculty was localized.[9] Both these doctrines were, however, subordinate to the basic axiom that "the brain constitutes an indispensable condition for the manifestation [of the mental faculties], it is their seat."[10]

A later, last-ditch effort to turn back the localizationist tide occurred at the 1881 International Medical Congress in London. There the German physiologist Friedrich Goltz (1834–1902) challenged the experimental

---

[5] "Discussion," pp. 580–581.
[6] Ibid., p. 582.
[7] Ibid., p. 594.
[8] Ibid.
[9] Ibid., p. 587.
[10] Ibid., p. 636.

basis of David Ferrier's theory of cortical localization.[11] The debate over the dog displayed by Goltz and the two monkeys exhibited by Ferrier was represented as "a Homeric contest of transcendent moment to the advancement of knowledge, and vital to the interests of mankind." The issue was finally decided in Ferrier's favour effectively sealing the orthodoxy of his position; as the narrator put it, "now all doubt as to the truth of the great doctrine of cerebral localisation was put to rest, and the ground prepared for the immense progress of the coming years."[12]

The localizationist orthodoxy both constrained and enabled particular modes of talking and writing about mind and brain. These activities formed part of a wider program of scientific work. Bouillaud's second axiom was, in particular, tantamount to an invitation, if not an injunction, to fill the cognitive blanks of cerebral space by apportioning certain parts of mind to determinate locations in the brain. In the second half of the nineteenth century clinicians and physiologists throughout Europe as well as elsewhere in the Western world took up this challenge. The cerebral conditions of language became their special concern.

This chapter is concerned with the unfolding of the discourse of aphasia in the period from 1861 to around 1900. It seeks to show, in particular, how certain forms of utterance and textual performance were endowed with a privileged and mandatory status within this endeavor while others were excluded or merely neglected. Its subject is, in other words, what Foucault calls the "internal régime of power"[13] that structured the practice and productions of aphasiology.

Building an Archive

In 1889 the American physician M. Allen Starr wrote: "There is no subject in the domain of medical science which enforces more strongly the necessity of following closely the inductive method of reasoning than this one of cerebral localization. The conclusions thus far arrived at have been reached by the collection and analysis of facts."[14] The passage rehearses a

---

[11] "Discussion on the Localization of Function in the Cortex Cerebri," *Transactions of the International Medical Congress*, 4 vols. (London: J. W. Kolckmann, 1881), vol. 1, pp. 218–241.

[12] Charles A. Ballance, *A Glimpse into the History of the Surgery of the Brain* (London: Macmillan, 1922), pp. 89–90.

[13] Michel Foucault, "Truth and Power," in *Power/Knowledge: Selected Interviews and Other Writings 1972–1977*, ed. Colin Gordon. (New York: Pantheon Books, 1980), p. 112.

[14] M. Allen Starr, "Aphasia," *Transactions of the Congress of American Physicians and Surgeons* 1 (1889): p. 879.

number of familiar empiricist tropes. But it also expresses the power exerted by a particular conception of progress in medical science. Taking the methodology of "inductive science" as a model, the motor for medical advance was construed as the accumulation of an ever greater number of relevant "facts." These facts could, moreover, be derived from only one source:

> Physiology had, it is true, shown the way; it had led up to an hypothesis regarding cerebral action in man. But the conclusions on which we rely have been derived almost wholly from the comparison of large numbers of clinical cases, supplemented by pathological records. And every decided advance in the knowledge of the localization of functions has been due to the careful collation of cases with autopsies and the study of their common features.[15]

Earlier in the same passage Starr had reinforced the sense of an obligation upon clinicians to contribute to the localizationist undertaking when he declared that the "*responsibility* for further progress rests, therefore, with physicians." [Italics added.] From the mid-nineteenth century medical men had striven to fulfil this obligation by turning their encounters with patients to scientific use.

Among the first to turn the clinical gaze in a systematic way upon those suffering from speech loss was the Parisian physician Armand Trousseau (1801–67). Although not a specialist in the diseases of the nervous system, after 1861 Trousseau paid particular attention to such cases when they appeared on his wards at the Hôtel-Dieu. Thus "the woman Desteben," whose symptoms included loss of speech, was "the object of our closest attention, and each day we spent a lot of time by her bed."[16] The use of the first person plural was not merely an token of Trousseau's sense of self-importance, but was indicative of the collective nature of the investigative enterprise in which he was engaged. Not only he but also his students became engrossed in the emergent science of aphasiology. At one of his clinical lectures on the case of another aphasic, who had stayed a full year at the Hôtel-Dieu, Trousseau reminded them of "the long sessions we have spent around her bed to assure ourselves of the state of her intelligence."[17]

Patients might be offered as gifts by colleagues anxious to advance the cause of science. Because a sixty-year-old man in the care of another member of the medical staff at the Hôtel-Dieu displayed "the most clear symp-

---

[15] Ibid.

[16] A. Trousseau, *Clinique médicale de l'Hôtel-Dieu de Paris* (Paris: Baillière, 1865), p. 572.

[17] Ibid., p. 587.

toms of aphasia," the physician concerned hastened to refer him to Trousseau's attention. When a case was regarded as especially "interesting" other senior members of the profession might be invited to join the process of contemplation and examination. In this instance Broca himself was asked to attend the autopsy which was conducted in his presence "with the greatest care."[18] Such ritualistic practices helped to reinforce the existence and solidarity of a community of workers devoted to a shared way of life. The iconic status that Broca had already acquired within aphasiology is also noteworthy.

It was understandable that the project of aphasiology should first take root in Paris. But the endeavor rapidly spread to Britain; the existence of a well-developed international medical press facilitated the rapid dissemination of the new sense of responsibility. In Germany, on the other hand, there was intitial resistance to the aphasiological enterprise although this was overcome by the 1870s.[19]

Practitioners in other countries began to follow James Russell's example by examining their "casebooks" to find instances relevant to the concerns of the new science.[20] From this it was a short step to seeking and recording new cases which in an earlier era might have suffered oblivion. In 1866 William Rutherford Sanders, one of the physicians at the Royal Infirmary of Edinburgh, published what he claimed was "the first case [of aphasia] completed by an autopsy which has occurred in Great Britain since attention has lately been directed to the subject by the French observers." Sanders' case appeared to corroborate Broca's hypothesis. It would, he conceded,

> be an absurdity in science to lay much weight on any coincidence, however extraordinary, and I should not be hasty to draw conclusions from the case just narrated. But it is evident that the questions of cerebral action, in relation to speech, have reached that stage in which definite observations are attainable, either in support or refutation of professed opinions.[21]

---

[18] Ibid., p. 592. More than thirty years later the practice of cultivating an "interesting" case by multiplying the number of practitioners involved in its study and demonstrating it to students was still current. See: H. Charlton Bastian, "On a Case of Amnesia and other Speech Defects of Eighteen Years' Duration with Autopsy," *Medico-Chirurgical Transactions* 18 (1897): 61–86, p. 62.

[19] See: Michael Hagner, "Aspects of Brain Localization in Late XIXth Century Germany," in Claude Debru (ed.), *Essays in the History of the Physiological Sciences* (Amsterdam: Clio Medical No. 33), pp.75–78.

[20] James Russell, "Hemiplegia of the Right Side, with Loss of Speech," *British Medical Journal* 2 (1864): 81–85, 211–213, 239–241, 408–411, 619–621, p. 81.

[21] William R. Sanders, "Case illustrating the Supposed Connexion of Aphasia (Loss of the Cerebral Faculty of Speech) with Right Hemiplegia, and Lesion of the External Left Frontal Convolution of the Brain," *Edinburgh Medical Journal* 11 (1866): 811–823, p. 822.

In other words, while Broca may have given an initial impetus to the project of mapping the relations of language and the brain, the validity of aphasiology was no longer dependent upon the truth of his theory. Indeed, the refutation or at least qualification of Broca's original claim might prove to be as, if not more, productive endeavors.

A year after Sanders' initial investigations another Scottish practitioner published a more extensive contribution to the question of "The Pathology of Aphasia." Alexander Robertson's report showed that the same kind of careful cultivation of aphasic patients that Trousseau practised in Paris was now occurring even in such lesser centres as Glasgow. "Full reports of all the symptoms," Robertson insisted, "were taken by myself at the bedsides of the patients." Robertson's investigations were framed, in particular, "so as to ascertain as correctly as possible the condition of the mental powers generally, but more especially that of the reasoning faculty" in the cases in question.[22]

The compilation of such "full reports" became a characteristic, almost a fetish, of aphasiology. Among the imperative aspects of the discourse—and perhaps a clue to its success—was that it *made work* for those involved in its elaboration. From an early stage, the pioneers of the field insisted upon the exhaustive procedures that must be followed in the clinic in order to generate facts that might qualify as valid contributions. These demands were sometimes coupled with warnings about the possible pitfalls facing those engaged in this kind of enquiry. Trousseau advised his students that: "It is important to investigate whether *intelligence is impaired* in cases of aphasia, and to what extent it may be [affected]." It was, however, no easy matter to satisfy this desideratum:

> To evaluate the intelligence of aphasics we have only facial expression, writing and gesture. The expression . . . does not deviate much from the normal state, and, for this reason, it seems that the intelligence is sound; but here I will make an observation. You may have often found yourself talking to a dog and in a way to question it. You have assuredly then been struck by the clarity of its gaze, by the liveliness of the singular intelligence that shines from the animal's features; by the movements of its head, and often by the little cries, the accentuated growlings with which it accompanies these actions. You are surprised to be chatting with him, and how often does one say: "All that he lacks is speech." Ah well gentlemen! Apply this observation to the aphasic patient, and you will be persuaded that the facial expression is more vacant than that of the dog; and one will then agree that we need a few more signs in order to judge the intelligence of a man.[23]

[22] Alexander Robertson, "The Pathology of Aphasia," *Journal of Mental Science* 12 (1867): 503–521, pp. 503, 506.

[23] Trousseau, *Clinique médicale*, pp. 610–611.

Trousseau therefore underlined the difficulties confronting the student of aphasia, the complexities and obscurity of the problem that he essayed. But thereby he multiplied the amount of clinical work incumbent upon the student of aphasiology: a battery of tests was needed to make an accurate evaluation of any given case. He may also have hinted at the necessary exercise of an incommunicable clinical "tact" at the patient's bedside to obviate the uncertainties inherent in any diagnosis.

Later formulations of the workload of the aphasiologist tended, in contrast, to minimize such hermeneutic difficulties. They gave the impression that so long as the clinician was faithful to the standardized protocols of inquiry available, he would be able to perform the tasks assigned him by the discourse of which he was part. These procedures were even susceptible of textbook exposition. While Trousseau represented an early pioneering stage in the development of aphasia studies, these later texts are indicative of an emergent stage in the discourse where automation and replicability were valued more highly than personal virtuosity.

H. Charlton Bastian's *Treatise on Aphasia and Other Speech Defects* (1898) supplied a "Schema for the Examination of Aphasic and Amnesic Patients." This embodied the procedures employed for many years on the wards of University College Hospital in London. The schema consisted of thirty-four questions and procedures that the clinician confronted with an aphasic patient should ask and perform. Bastian also provided a table by means of which the physician would be able to infer from the "clinical characters" his investigations had revealed both the name of the speech defect with which he was presented as well as the site and nature of the lesion responsible for the symptoms (fig. 3.1).[24] Such devices putatively served to make diagnosis more mechanical and therefore more standardized; results obtained by these means were readily transported between workers in the same institution as well as around the aphasiological network.

The records of the National Hospital for Nervous Diseases in Queen's Square London show that from at least the 1870s attempts were made to conform to these protocols when dealing with patients with disordered language. Standard tests were scrupulously applied to ascertain an individual's speech, reading, and writing capacities in accordance with a prior categorization of these faculties and of the defects to which they were

---

[24] H. Charlton Bastian, *A Treatise on Aphasia and Other Speech Defects* (London: H.K. Lewis, 1898), pp. 307–311. For a somewhat shorter protocol for the clinical investigation of aphasia see: Starr, "Aphasia," p. 337. Such systems were the forerunners of later sets of test "batteries" to be applied rigorously to all cases of language loss. Henry Head's and Kurt Goldstein's contributions to the creation of such technologies are described elsewhere in this volume. Contemporary neurology has resort to such standardized diagnostic resources as the Boston Assessment of Severe Aphasia and similar systems.

THE CLINICAL CHARACTERISTICS, TOGETHER WITH THE SITES IN WHICH LESIONS ARE TO BE LOOKED FOR, OF DIFFERENT FORMS OF SPEECH DEFECT.

Name of Speech Defect.	Its Clinical Characters.	Site and Nature of Lesion.
1. ANARTHRIA.	Defective power of articulation —speech more or less unintelligible. Mind clear — understands all that is said to him. Can express himself freely by writing, when hand not paralysed. Will attempt to repeat any word when bidden to do so. There is commonly difficulty in deglutition, and there may be more or less bilateral paralysis of limbs.[1]	*Damage to Bulbar Speech Centres.*
2. APHEMIA.	(*a*) *Complete.* Patient is absolutely dumb. Mind clear and understands everything said to him. Writes freely and correctly when not paralysed on the right side (Cases xi., xii.). (*b*) *Incomplete.* Articulation more or less defective, but no tendency to use wrong words. Understands everything that is said to him. Will attempt to repeat any word when bidden to do so. Can write freely and correctly, when not paralysed on the right side.	*Damage to Efferent Fibres from Broca's Centre.*
3. APHASIA.	(*a*) Patient may be completely dumb. Mind clear, and understands everything said to him. Will not attempt to repeat any word. Can write freely and correctly, when not paralysed on the right side.	*Due either* (1) *to Functional Defects in both Third Frontal Convolutions (Hysterical Mutism); or* (2) *to an Organic Lesion absolutely limited to Broca's Centre (Case* xxii.*).*

Figure 3.1. Schema for examination of aphasic and amnesiac patients. H. Charlton Bastian, *Treatise on Aphasia and Other Speech Defects* (1898)

susceptible.[25] Bastian attempted to impose these procedures upon future generations of medical practitioners by means of his clinical lectures at University College Hospital.[26]

In mature products of the aphasiological discourse produced during the 1880s and 1890s inscriptions produced by such methods featured prominently in published research papers. It was common practice to print extensive transcripts of the patient's attempts at speech and writing. Facsimiles of the aphasic's own hand were sometimes also reproduced in an effort to delimit the nature and extent of the lesion to written language in a given case.[27] Conversely, Jean Martin Charcot (1825–93) generated tables recording the time it took a patient to read a given text over the course of his illness.[28]

The emphasis here was upon the degree of *certainty* to which the clinical method could aspire provided that its practitioners were properly disciplined. Individual clinical skill was esteemed less than a readiness to acquiesce in one's labors to a schema imposed as it were from above. Indeed, individuality was figured as a source of error to be eliminated as far as was possible. The desiderata were results amenable to comparison, collation, and ultimate incorporation into a case archive available to all aphasiology.

Although clinicians were the most obvious authors of this archive, patients also necessarily played a crucial role in its production. The patient sometimes figured merely as an animalized or even reified object of medical contemplation or manipulation. William Henry Broadbent, in an analogy reminiscent of Trousseau, recorded his impressions of one case as: "Face intelligent, eyes bright, and remind one of an intelligent dog from the keen way in which he watches one's face and movements."[29]

James Russell's case histories showed even less trace of any human identification with the patient. He wrote of one patient that:

> it was impossible to elicit any evidence of common sensation; most severe pinching, pushing the point of a knife into his skin, the application of a spoon dipped in boiling water, pulling his whiskers, thrusting a pin behind the fin-

---

[25] This is evident in the clinical records of the National Hospital for Nervous Diseases in Queen's Square London: see, e.g., Bastian's Casebook for 1879, pp. 5–12, 215.

[26] W. D. Halliburton, [Clinical Lectures at University College Hospital by H. Charlton Bastian, October 1882], Wellcome Institute for the History of Medicine MS 2705, pp. 256–257.

[27] See, for example, M. J. Dejerine, "Contribution à l'étude des troubles de l'écriture chez les aphasiques," *Comptes rendus des séances et mémoires de la Société de Biologie* 43 (1891): 97–113, pp. 101–108.

[28] [Jean Martin] Charcot, "Des différentes formes de l'aphasie.—De la cécité verbale," *Le progrès médicale* 11 (1883): p. 443.

[29] William Henry Broadbent, "On the Cerebral Mechanism of Speech and Thought," *Medico-Chirurgical Transactions* 55 (1872): 145–194, p. 156.

ger nail, produced no sign of sensibility—not the least change in the face—
nothing, in short, but a few inconsiderable muscular movements in the limb
which was assailed.

Russell himself described such procedures as "tortures."[30]

But the creation of an aphasiology required a more varied and dynamic
contribution from patients. The "typical" aphasic was no mere passive
body bereft of all capacity for response and spontaneity; he or she took an
active role in the generation of the case history. The character of that
contribution was, however, constrained. "Nothing," Sanders insisted,

> is more evident than that the patient thinks, and that he is extremely anxious
> to communicate his thoughts. His face and eyes appear full of expression, and
> he makes eager efforts to convey his meaning, and, when he fails, he betrays
> his disappointment, according to the nature of his disposition, either by a
> good-natured smile and laugh, or else by frowns and tears.[31]

The nature of the patient's contribution to the case was determined by
the extent of the character of his or her lesion of language; indeed, the
whole point of the exercise was to ascertain the character of that deficit.
But even when a patient was utterly speechless, he or she could still, Charcot maintained, provide an "animated pantomime" for the edification of
his medical audience; by means of such mime it was possible to determine,
for instance, whether or not the identity and use of common objects were
still recognised. Moreover, this kind of dumb show might even be accompanied by a musical interlude: Charcot noted that a certain patient was
still capable of giving a rendering of the "Marseillaise."[32] One of Joseph
Jules Dejerine's patients was yet more talented, singing "very correctly
various operatic pieces."[33]

When speech was only impaired rather than suppressed the patient's
repertoire as a performer was greatly enhanced. A case recounted by the
Manchester physician James Ross in 1887 more closely resembled a music-
hall turn than an operatic recital. The patient in question was "always an
unsteady man, and his employment, in serving writs for the last few years,
favoured his drinking propensities, and he was a well-known character in
all the beer-houses in Manchester and neighbourhood." After a series of
fits the man's speech became became "incorrect."[34]

---

[30] Russell, "Hemiplegia," pp. 409–410.

[31] Sanders, "Case," p. 812.

[32] Charcot, "Des différentes formes," pp. 522–523.

[33] J. J. Dejerine, "Différentes variétés de cécité verbale," *Comptes rendus des séances et mémoires de la Société de Biologie* 44 (1892): 61–90, p. 74.

[34] James Ross, *On Aphasia: Being a Contribution to the Subject of the Dissolution of Speech from Cerebral Disease* (London: J. & A. Churchill, 1887), p. 30.

In the clinic protracted efforts were made to establish the character of his linguistic disorder:

> He was now handed a bunch of keys, and asked to name one of them. He held one between his thumb and index finger, and said, "It is a public-house." "That is not a public-house," I said. "I know it quite well;" he replied, "I have seen it thousands of times," and, trying again to name it, he continued, "It is a—it is a public-house. Pooh! I know it quite well.[35]

Later the report notes the "comical expression" the patient's face assumed as he continued in his efforts to name various items. Ross went on to provide a further "very laughable illustration of the manner in which he used the word 'public-house' on all occasions." The patient's attempts at writing were likewise "somewhat ludicrous"—a point illustrated by a facsimile.[36] Such risible behavior was not, however, incorrigible. The report noted that after several years of such repartee, it had been possible to "reorganis[e] in him the names of common objects." One result of these training exercises was that his previous "comical expression" was now replaced by an "intelligent smile."[37]

Bouillaud in 1865 was already able to describe the as yet rudimentary aphasia archive as "this *levée en masse*, this army of facts."[38] Within a few years aphasiologists were in a position to inspect, marshal, and regiment this army in order to fight a variety of theoretical battles. A "secondary, complex" literary genre arose which employed case histories as its primary material.[39] In the process, the relations of that raw or semiprocessed matter changed: the immediate referents of the clinical narrative came to count for less than their alleged universal significance.[40] To pursue Bouillaud's metaphor, the discrete combatants of the aphasiological army became subsumed within the larger formations of which they formed the basic element. As in war, the individual soldier was expendable.

In his 1869 discussion of aphasia Frederic Bateman made reference to no fewer than seventy-two cases in the course of his argument. He also

---

[35] Ibid., p. 31.

[36] Ibid., pp. 31–33.

[37] Ibid., pp. 36–37.

[38] "Discussion," p. 623.

[39] For the distinction between primary and secondary genres see: M. M. Bakhtin, "The Problem of Speech Genres," in *Speech Genres and Other Late Essays*, trans. Vern W. McGee, (Austin: University of Texas Press, 1986), pp. 60–102, on p. 62.

[40] To adapt Bakhtin's terms once more, this shift might be characterized as one marked by the emergence of a new *addressee*—or perhaps *superaddressee*—for these utterances ("The Problem of the Text," ibid., pp. 103–131, pp. 98, 126). Rather than any empirical collection of readers or assessors, the true audience becomes the particular refraction of an abstract scientific subjectivity.

tried to sketch the heuristic rules to be employed in future exercises of this sort. He identified a "common error into which many observers fall": namely, the tendency "to confine their attention to the consideration of typical cases only . . . ; whereas, as much or more information may sometimes be gained from the careful study of exceptional cases."[41]

The cases Bateman mustered according to these principles served as so many witnesses for and against the various hypotheses that had been advanced on the relation of language to the brain. His estimation of Broca's theory, for instance, consisted both of a critical reading of the case of "Tan" and an exposition of some of Bateman's own more recent clinical records. Both procedures tended to invalidate Broca's localization of the seat of language in the third frontal convolution of the left hemisphere.[42]

This dual strategy became extremely characteristic of later aphasiology. At the same time as "modern" cases were presented for the first time, the texts of old, "classic" cases were subjected to close exegesis often leading to novel readings that diverged from that of their authors.[43] Within the course of a career it was even possible for the same author to arrive at discrepant readings of a particular case.[44]

Such divergent interpretation of texts and disagreements over the theoretical bearing of cases was not viewed as a reproach or embarrassment to the aphasiological project. On the contrary, the discourse generated rhetorical resources that made such vacillation appear a virtue. In Bastian's formulation there was a necessary dialectic between hypotheses and the clinical facts that could alone validate or undermine them.[45] As more cases were added to the archive so the theoretical structure of aphasiology must necessarily change. At the same time older cases would be read in the fresh light shed by more modern concepts. By means of these maneuvers both the inherently progressive nature of the aphasiologists' endeavor and the epistemological primacy of the contents of the clinical archive were safeguarded.

[41] Frederic Bateman, "On Aphasia or Loss of Speech in Cerebral Disease," *Journal of Mental Science* 14 (1869): 50–74, 345–365, 489–504, p. 346.

[42] Frederic Bateman, "Aphasia or Loss of Speech in Cerebral Disease," *Journal of Mental Science* 15 (1870): 102–119, 367–393, pp. 377–378.

[43] See, for instance, Bastian's reinterpretation of cases of Trousseau and Lichtheim bearing on the question of alexia: H. Charlton Bastian, "Some Problems in Connexion with Aphasia and other Speech Defects," *Lancet* 1 (1897): 933–942, 1005–1017, 1131–1137, 1187–1194, pp. 1009–1010. On the role of classic texts in the development of a scientific specialty see: Gyorgy Markus, "Why is there no Hermeneutics of Natural Sciences?: Some Preliminary Theses," *Science in Context* 1 (1987): 5–51, p. 35.

[44] Bastian, "Some Problems," p. 1188.

[45] Ibid., p. 1131.

The Classificatory Imperative

The privileged status of the "facts" embodied in case histories was too fundamental a tenet ever to be questioned. But protests against an excessively slavish adherence to the rhetoric of empiricism were heard from an early stage in the history of aphasiology. Thus Henry Maudsley in 1868 had already declared that "inquiry into this obscure subject has arrived at a stage when little or no further profit can accrue from an aimless accumulation of observations, and that what now is needed is a digestion of the material which lies at hand."[46] This process of digestion required ordering the word heap of the archive according to some principle of subordination and relation.

The most obvious response to this program was to attempt some classification of cases on a symptomological basis. Even in the mid-nineteenth century the spirit of nosology was far from dead. Trousseau in his clinical lectures distinguished between various "species" of aphasia on the basis of whether or not intelligence was affected.[47] Others, such as Jules-Gabriel-François Baillarger, preferred to distinguish between cases of "simple" aphasia in which the power to translate ideas into words was lost and those where words were used to express ideas, but incorrectly.[48]

Bastian in 1869 went beyond these simple binary divisions to create a more elaborate, although still comparatively rudimentary, branching system in which the general order of "Loss of Speech" was successively divided into different genera, species, and varieties.[49] One purpose served by Bastian's classification was to distinguish "true" aphasia from various other aphonic conditions.

Although Bastian's taxonomic efforts were symptomatic of aphasiologists' attempts to impose an order upon the ever growing number of cases in the archive, no consensus emerged. Different authors deemed various and incompatible systems to be the most simple, convenient, compelling, or "natural."[50] Nor was there any agreement on matters of terminology: even the basal category "aphasia" was variously construed as either generic or as only applicable to certain specific kinds of speech disorder.

Despite this diversity, all these classificatory systems were derived from comparable cultural materials: namely, conventional nineteenth-century

---

[46] Henry Maudsley, "Concerning Aphasia," *Lancet* 2 (1868): 690–692, 721–723, p. 690.

[47] Trousseau, *Clinique médicale*, p. 615.

[48] "Discussion," p. 618.

[49] H. Charlton Bastian, "On the Various Forms of Loss of Speech in Cerebral Disease," *British and Foreign Medico-Chirurgical Review* 43 (1869): 209–236, 470–492, p. 211.

[50] For a review of the various classifications thrown up in the early years of aphasiology see: Bateman, "On Aphasia" (1869), pp. 494–495.

notions of the nature of normal language and its relation to mind. Henry Maudsley was unusually clear in his appreciation of how these tacit assumptions informed—and, in *his* view, distorted—the views of his contemporaries. Such a conflation of psychology and medicine was unavoidable given the nature of the subject; the consideration of language, Maudsley maintained,

> brings us at once to that unknown region which lies between what we call mind and what we call matter—to that great barrier which man, having himself first set it up, has been occupied generation after generation in adding to, lamenting all the while that he can find no means of passing it. On the one hand, language is in the most intimate relation with the operations of mind, having, indeed, an essential part in them; on the other hand, it is a mode of physical expression. . . . Between the thought of the mind and the word which is the sign or utterance of the thought lies that great gulf which no one has yet fathomed or thrown a bridge across.[51]

But what Maudlsey did censure was the casual and uncritical way in which aphasiologists had employed psychological terms in their efforts to lay at least the foundations of such a bridge. "Had the subjective method been properly used," he insisted, "and the psychological relations of language duly considered, it may be questioned whether the theory that a part of the third left frontal convolution was the seat of articulate language would ever have been promulgated so hastily, and, I may add, received so rashly." In Maudsley's view, "there has been nothing like it in psychology since Descartes located the soul in the pineal gland."[52]

Maudsley held that the very notion of a "faculty of speech" that might be located in this or that part of the brain was flawed. Broca and those who followed him had, in effect, been deceived by a "wonderful metaphysical entity, distinct from the phenomena"; the worth of all their clinical labours was therefore vitiated.[53] Maudsley did not aim to undermine the project of aphasiology as such; but he did insist upon the need for a critical attitude to the psychological categories that must by the nature of the exercise be employed in this endeavour. He thus anticipated the strictures of such later critics as Henry Head upon aspects of the classic aphasiological project (see chapter 5).

Maudsley's colleagues were, however, more conventional than critical in their use of psychological concepts. In Britain clinicians like Bastian simply took over the dominant associationist model of the mental opera-

---

[51] Maudlsey, "On Aphasia," p. 690.
[52] Ibid., pp. 690–691.
[53] Ibid., p. 692.

tions underlying the origin and operations of language.[54] The various forms of diseased language were then figured in terms of a breakdown of some part of the mechanism of normal speech, reading, and writing.[55]

Charcot too found the doctrines of the "great English school" of psychology serviceable enough in his own clinical writings;[56] he implied, however, that these theories merely confirmed facts about the nature of language that had emerged in an unmediated way from clinical experience. Both sources agreed that words consisted of four "elements or factors": namely, the auditory, visual, and the two forms of motor "image" corresponding to speech and writing respectively.[57] These elements were variously combined in the constitution of any individual. In a manner akin to the old humoral physiology, Charcot maintained that certain factors tended to predominate in particular types of person: thus there were *visuels* and *auditifs*, *moteurs graphiques* as well as *moteurs d'articulation*; others, however, in whom there was a balance between these sensory and motor elements, were merely *indifférents*.[58]

The existence of this common syntax did much to counteract the tendency to dissolution evident in the early attempts at classification in aphasiology. Indeed, the associationist model provided a common language within which disputation about matters of taxonomic detail could occur.

In moving beyond mere tabular classification towards the use of models that purported to explain the dynamics of normal and pathological language aphasiology conceded that the clinical gaze alone was inadequate to a proper ordering of the phenomenon in question. Another kind of imagination, one that transcended words themselves, was required before the keystone of Maudsley's imaginary bridge could be laid.

Disciplinary Designs

Writing in 1874, some ten years after the inception of the project of aphasiology, Carl Wernicke outlined certain shortcomings of the by now volu-

---

[54] See: H. Charlton Bastian, "On the Physiology of Thinking," *Fortnightly Review* 5n.s. (1869): 57–71.

[55] Bastian, "On Aphasia," pp. 216–217.

[56] Charcot's choice of phrase is probably an allusion to the positivist philosopher Théodule Ribot's attempts to introduce French readers to "la psychologie anglaise contemporaine." See: John I. Brooks, *The Eclectic Legacy: Academic Philosophy and the Human Sciences in Nineteenth-Century France* (Newark: University of Delaware Press, 1998), p. 71.

[57] Pierre Marie, "De l'aphasie en général et de l'agraphie en particulier, d'après l'enseignement de M. le professeur Charcot," *Le Progrès Médicale* 7 second series (1888): 81–84, pp. 81–82.

[58] Ibid., p. 83.

minous archive of case histories produced by workers in the field. "The clinical aphasia literature [*Casuistik der Aphasie*]," he complained,

> rich as it may be, is of limited value for the support of any kind of anatomi-cally-based theory. This is in part a reflection of the subjective nature of case interpretations supplied by most examiners. For example, in various case histories published by a single observer, the major emphasis is usually on one new, unique symptom, not previously reported in the literature. The complete psychic symptomatology, however, is neglected. Or, avoiding this error, we may find tedious, detailed, but objective reports with omission of the most important information.

One desideratum was thus the elimination of the subjective in writing on aphasia along with the pursuit of an ideal objectivity.

Existing accounts were inadequate because they failed to supply the detailed investigation of "psychic symptom complexes" demanded by the kind of theoretical discourse which Wernicke proposed.[59] The passage makes clear that Wernicke's perceived problem was disciplinary in nature—taking full account of the ambiguities of the term.[60] In order to create an adequate (i.e., theoretical) discipline of aphasiology, it was necessary to discipline the labours of those generating foundational clinical studies. The "raw" materials of aphasia studies needed, in fact, to be to some degree preprocessed if they were to meet Wernicke's criteria of serviceability.

He also specified that the discipline he sought to establish was to be particularly concerned with the "anatomical relations" of the subject. This might at first sight appear a weak and unexceptional stipulation: clinical observation had, from Bouillaud's early inquiries onwards, been supplemented by attempts to localize at autopsy the lesions responsible for any given set of symptoms. On the basis of such postmortem investigations, conclusions had been drawn as to the "seat" of language or of some component part of that faculty.

These previous pathological efforts were, however, also flawed; this was the second "evil" [*Übelstand*] besetting aphasiology. The evil did not derive from any lack of skills among those engaged in this inquiry. There

---

[59] Carl Wernicke, "The Aphasia Symptom Complex: A Psychological Study on an Anatomical Basis," in Gertrude H. Eggert, *Wernicke's Works on Aphasia: A Sourcebook and Review* (The Hague: Mouton, 1977), p. 118 (38). This is a translation of Wernicke's *Der aphasische Symptomencomplex: Eine psychologische Studie auf anatomischer Basis* (Breslau: Max Cohn & Weigert, 1874). I have occasionally modified Eggert's translation. Numerals in parentheses in this and subsequent citations refer to the pages of the original German text.

[60] On the various productive ambiguities of the term see: Jan Goldstein, "Foucault among the Sociologists: The 'Disciplines' and the History of the Professions," *History and Theory* 23 (1984): 170–192, especially pp. 178–179.

was no question but that Broca, John Hughlings Jackson, and the other "most important authors on aphasia," were sufficiently "experienced" neuroanatomists to give accurate and trustworthy reports of the lesions they discovered at autopsy.[61] But because of the inadequacies of the materials with which they worked the results attained were ambivalent; in this department of aphasiological work too there was therefore a need for greater discipline.

Wernicke articulated a set of convictions inherent in earlier expositions of the aphasiological program. Clinical description was seen as merely the first step; even when accompanied by a classification of cases according to some psychological schema, aphasiology must ultimately be grounded upon a somatic basis. The ultimate referent of its discourse was the brain. More specifically, aphasiology was concerned with events occurring on and within the cortex of the cerebral hemispheres.

A precondition of such discourse was the construction of *the* brain as a natural object. The definite article implied a generic entity of which all empirical brains were particular manifestations.[62] In the case of the cerebral cortex this unifying entity came into being only in the mid-nineteenth century. Whereas earlier observers had seen only chaos in the convolutions, comparing them to the random windings of the intestines, after 1800 a novel uniformity was discerned in these structures.[63] The result of this development was the emergence of representations of *the* cerebral cortex, an object providing a template for the contemplation of any individual brain.[64]

By the 1860s this template had become a necessary adjunct to the pathological explication of a given case. Before describing the extent of a particular lesion it was, Trousseau insisted, needful, "briefly to recall the disposition and the relations of the cerebral organs which should be mentioned in the description of the lesion." He proceeded to supply a verbal mapping of the area bounded by the sylvian and rolandic fissures relying for the most part on Broca's account of this region of the cortex.[65]

---

[61] Wernicke, "Aphasia Symptom Complex," pp. 118–119 (38).

[62] Cf. Nietzsche's discussion of the formulation of the idea of *the* primal "leaf." "On Truth and Falsity in their Ultramoral Sense," *The Complete Works of Friedrich Nietzsche*, ed. Oscar Levy (London: Allen and Unwin, 1911), vol. 2, pp. 173–192, on p. 179.

[63] The most authoritative of these schema is found in: Pierre Gratiolet, *Mémoire sur les plis cérébraux de l'homme et des primates* (Paris: Arthur Bertrand, 1854).

[64] Depictions of the cortex were therefore images of a "typical" object. The history of the visual imagery employed in neurology and neurophysiology does not accord well with the secular tendency *away* from such representations of the type of a natural object that Lorraine Daston and Peter Galison have discerned: "The Image of Objectivity," *Representations* 40 (1992): 81–128.

[65] Trousseau, *Clinique médicale*, pp. 598–599.

This word map was taken up by other authors seeking a common terrain on which to locate their observations. National boundaries proved no obstacle to its dissemination. "The minute anatomy of the brain not being to my knowledge described in any English author with the same amount of detail as occurs in M. Broca's description," Frederic Bateman conceded, "I have condensed the following account from his work, 'Sur le Siège de la Faculté du Langage Articulé.' "[66]

But Bateman was not content merely to copy Broca's words; he also reproduced an engraving of the left cerebral hemisphere, "shewing the disposition and arrangement of the cerebral convolutions, from a cast kindly sent to the author by Prof. Broca of Paris."[67] The engraving in question aspired to a naturalistic particularity: an attempt was made to convey the contours and shadowing of the surface of the brain. But features deemed significant were labelled by means of numbers and letters which referred to an accompanying key (see fig. 3.2). These marks signified aspects of the ideal, universal cortex.

By despatching representations of this structure throughout the nascent aphasiological network, Broca was ensuring that there would be a common surface on which to plot the anatomical correlates of speech disorder. Even among the foot soldiers of the new science there was, moreover, an awareness of the necessity of an agreed terminology and visual language. Sanders in 1866 expressed this as an imperative: "The post-mortem examinations of the surface of the brain must in future be made with great accuracy, in reference to the systems of convolutions on the basis of Gratiolet's classification."[68] As an exemplar he cited a recent article on the degeneration of the cerebrum by Kenneth M'Leod in which description of postmortem appearances was regulated by "the system and nomenclature of Gratiolet."[69]

In the accompanying illustrations M'Leod continued to employ techniques of stippling and shading in order to give an illusion of three dimensionality. Parts of the brain were, moreover, depicted as cut away to suggest the interior depths of the structure. His engravings were of "brains" more than of the brain. The particularity of these instances of the structure was reinforced by scrupulous notation of the dimensions of each organ

---

[66] Frederic Bateman, "On Aphasia or Loss of Speech in Cerebral Disease," *Journal of Mental Science* 13 (1868): 521–532, p. 522.

[67] Frederic Bateman, *On Aphasia or Loss of Speech, and the Localisation of the Faculty of Articulate Language* (London: John Churchill, 1870), p. 392.

[68] Sanders, "Case," p. 822. Contributions which did not conform to "our present mode of dividing the brain" could be deemed invalid: Bateman, *On Aphasia*, p. 373.

[69] Kenneth M'Leod, "Case of Degeneration and Atrophy of the Cerebrum, Causing Unilateral Epilepsy," *Edinburgh Medical Journal* 10 (1865): 323–338, p. 330.

Engraving of the Convex Surface of the Left Hemisphere.

Showing the Disposition and Arrangement of the Cerebral Convolutions.

From a Cast kindly sent to the Author by his lamented friend, the late Professor Broca, of Paris.

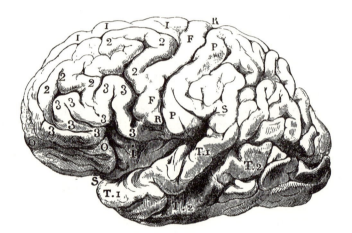

RR, Fissure of Rolando.

SS, Fissure of Sylvius.

1, 2, 3, First, second, and third frontal convolutions.

FF, Transverse frontal convolution.

PP, Transverse parietal convolution.

OO, Orbital convolutions.

T1, T2, First and second temporo-sphenoidal convolutions.

I, Island of Reil (the superior and inferior marginal convolutions are represented as being drawn asunder so as to expose it.)

Figure 3.2. Engraving of the convex surface of the left hemisphere.
Frederic Bateman, *On Aphasia* (1890)

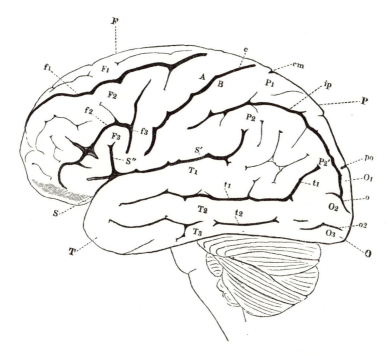

Figure 3.3. Lateral view of the human brain. David Ferrier,
The Functions of the Brain (1876)

depicted. The relation of these representations to Gratiolet's schema remained relatively loose and impressionistic.

This style of representation tended, however, to become superseded in
the aphasiological canon by more stereotyped, two-dimensional brain profiles. Such designs were more "schematic" not only because of their greater
simplicity and similarity, but also because the standard mapping of cortical
features was integral rather than accidental to their composition. Illustrative devices of this kind were generally deemed to have derived from the
work of "French authors"; but they rapidly attained international currency
(fig. 3.3). They constituted the basis of a shared visual language for the
aphasiological discipline.[70] Through such designs the brain was rendered
a more "docile" object.[71]

[70] Compare Martin Rudwick's discussion of the role of the creation of a shared visual
language in the disciplinary consolidation of geology: "The Emergence of a Visual Language
for Geological Science, 1760–1840," *History of Science* 14 (1976): 149–195, especially
p. 177.

[71] I take this term from: Michael Lynch, "Discipline and the Material Forms of Scientific
Visibility," *Social Studies of Science* 15 (1985): 37–66, p. 43.

The lectures that Charcot gave on the principles of cerebral localization in the 1880s illustrate how the authority of these disciplinary devices was inculcated into novice investigators through pedagogy. He insisted to his students upon the old phrenological notion that the brain was no "homogeneous, unitary organ, but indeed an association, or if you will a federation constituted by a certain number of separate organs."[72] The boundaries of the constituent parts of this federation were, moreover, determinate: the fixity of the "departments" distributed upon the surface of the brain was incontestable.[73] Nature had therefore provided a strategic map to which the clinician-pathologist must refer when engaged in his craft; he was to strive towards a *"regional diagnostics* of brain disease."[74]

Charcot instructed his students in what they should see as they dissected the brain. At the same time he imposed a nomenclature which constrained and disciplined the linguistic performances that accompanied such procedures. These strictures applied to the anatomy of the brain as a whole; however,

> The importance of an exact and minute study of the configuration of the divisions [*circonscriptions*] of the brain and . . . of an appropriate nomenclature, is above all evident when dealing with the folds outlined on the surface of the hemispheres, and which generally go under the name of *convolutions*.

Without "a good topography" of these structures, it was "entirely impossible to take a step in the narrative of the most important cerebral localizations."[75]

Illustrations played a crucial role in the pedagogic enforcement of the preferred cerebral topography. The primary subdivisions of the cortex were first demonstrated by reference to a picture of the simian brain; after

---

[72] J. M. Charcot, "De la localisation dans les maladies cérébrales," in *Oeuvres Complètes de J.M. Charcot* (Paris: A. Delamaye, 1887), vol. 4, p. 3.

[73] Ibid., p. 16.

[74] Ibid., p. 2. Charcot's use of political and administrative terms such as "federation" and "department" in his account of the project of mapping the "regions" of the brain disclosed, almost incidentally, the affinity between the project of cerebral localization and that of geography. In both instances mapping was instrumental to the exercise of particular forms of power. In the case of mapping the surface of the brain there is, first, an obvious claim to pedagogic authority of professor over student: the latter is to see the brain in accordance with the former's precepts. But in more circuitous ways the disease and the bearer of the disease are also disciplined by these maneuvers. See the suggestive remarks in Michel Foucault, "Questions on Geography," in *Power/Knowledge*, pp. 68–70. For a discussion of the links between geographic colonization and the "opening up" of the body see: Georg Stauth and Bryan S. Turner, *Nietzsche's Dance: Resentment, Reciprocity and Resistance in Social Life* (Oxford: Basil Blackwell, 1988), pp. 86–87.

[75] Ibid., p. 9.

this contemplation of the convolutions in the ape, Charcot insisted, that the study of "the corresponding convolutions in man becomes more simple. The enumeration I am about to make with the aid of a diagram . . . will make you easily recognize this truth."[76] Pictorial truth was thus deemed somehow more transparent and irrefragable than that propagated by mere words. It was thus a potent device in discipline formation.

Narrative Devices

Although "French" style brain profiles were highly schematic, they nonetheless purported to represent the essential features of a natural object available to sensory examination. But the discourse of aphasia became famous—in the eyes of some, infamous—for its attempts to achieve a higher degree of abstraction. After 1871, Henry Head maintained, "the rage for diagrams became a veritable mania."[77] In Head's retrospective view, the process of civilizing the brain had been taken too far by the early generation of aphasiologists.

Those engaged in this endeavor had supposed that speech and other linguistic behaviors were explicable in terms of the action and interaction of certain "centers," which, together with their commissural pathways, could be schematically represented upon an abstract surface. The auditory, visual, and motor memories of words were held to be stored in various "depots" in the brain from whence they were drawn in the acts of speaking, listening, reading, and writing. A circulation of stimulus and response existed between these verbal stores.[78] In Bastian's words,

> I am disposed to maintain that in speaking we exercise a power of voluntary recall over the words we wish to employ, evolving them out of the parts of the cerebral hemispheres which have acted as "Perceptive centres" for auditory impressions. Then, this Volition still continuing, its energy may be transmuted into a stimulus capable of bringing about an almost automatic act of

[76] Ibid., p. 14.

[77] Henry Head, "Aphasia: An Historical Review," *Brain* 43 (1920): 390–411, on p. 396. Many of these diagrams are reproduced in: François Moutier, *L'aphasie de Broca* (Paris: G. Steinthal, 1908), pp. 32–60.

[78] In resorting to such a schema aphasiology may have relied on assumptions of self-evidence deeply embodied in contemporary scientific culture. Michel Serres has maintained that models composed of the common elements of *reservoirs* and *circulation* were fundamental to "the entire set of interpretative organons in the nineteenth century." *Hermes: Literature, Science, Philosophy* (Baltimore: Johns Hopkins Press, 1989), p. 38. One obvious analogue is with the centers of production and distributive networks integral to the working of an industrial economy.

a complicated nature—namely, one calling into play that delicate combination of the many muscles of the larynx, tongue, palate, and lips which is required for the Articulation of the word thought of.[79]

Such expositions of the mechanism of language bore an obvious debt to associationist psychology. Bastian did not hesitate, moreover, to resort to the venerable method of introspection in order to confirm inferences derived from this source.[80] The conventional and widely disseminated character of these assumptions is indicated by the fact that Bastian published this exposition of the "Physiology of Thinking" in a nonprofessional periodical designed for the general educated public.

When he came to elaborate these views in more strictly professional contexts, however, Bastian acknowledged a need to effect a translation from such relatively untrammeled discussion of the operations of the "mind" and the newly constrained anatomy of the brain. He admitted ignorance of the actual location of the cerebral centers he had invoked or of the "definite routes" by which impressions reached them. Nevertheless, "We may be sure," he maintained, "that such centres do exist somewhere, and are in connection with afferent fibres, bringing them into connection with ganglionic masses, existing nearer the base of the brain and the medulla oblongata." It was also fair to suppose "abundant communications" existed between these centers.[81] The ostentatious use of such scientific terms as "afferent fibres" and "ganglionic masses" provided at least a tenuous link between the psychological and the anatomical.

Some reconciliation between the language of hypothetical psychological operations and the grammar of cerebral anatomy was seen as an important desideratum by later aphasiology. It was no explanation of a case, William Broadbent proclaimed in 1879, "to invent names more or less expressive of the derangements observed, or to describe them in psychological terminology. What is wanted is that the damage in the cell and fibre mechanism of speech, and of the mental operations concerned in speech, shall be specified." This came to be known as the "anatomical approach." The aphasiologist's problem derived from the fact that this "mechanism is . . . yet unknown."[82]

Aphasiology's solution to this dilemma took the form of the invention of a genre of brain or nerve fable. These narratives comprised elements drawn from various sources including psychology, cerebral anatomy, and experimental physiology, as well as what might be designated conjectural

[79] Bastian, "On the Physiology," p. 63.
[80] Ibid., p. 65.
[81] Bastian, "Various Forms," p. 477.
[82] W. H. Broadbent, "A Case of Peculiar Affection of Speech, with Commentary," *Brain* 1 (1879): 484–503. p. 490.

physiological-anatomy. The "hard" factual elements served both to camouflage the more "hypothetical" bits of the tale and to supply an embodiment for psychological categories.

These fables, moreover, did not consist of verbal representations alone. Broadbent undertook to provide a basal account of how groups of sensory and motor cells might become "educated" to perform certain roles under the direction of higher centres; "a diagram," he suggested, "may assist in rendering the idea more clear."[83]

Extending this model to the understanding of speech, it followed that "there will be somewhere or other in the higher centres a set of motor nerve-cells, from which will descend fibres to the nerve-nuclei of the thoracic muscles for the production of an expiatory current of air; others to the larynx for phonation; others, again, to the tongue and lips for articulation." Broadbent sought to qualify the airiness of "somewhere or other" by hinting that this center might lie in a determinate anatomical structure: the corpus striatum. Similarly, he ventured to suggest that the third frontal convolution was the " 'way out' for intellectual expression by speech, for words in relation to ideas." Conversely, the "infra-marginal gyrus of the fissure of Sylvius" was a plausible candidate for the post of auditory perceptive center.[84]

While a due relation between these two cerebral centers was necessary to "precise and orderly utterance," damage to this mechanism explained pathological speech. Once again, "for the sake of clearness we may . . . resort to a diagram." From this diagram it was, Broadbent maintained, possible to predict what form of language defect would result from a lesion at any given point in the imagined mechanism (fig. 3.4). He took care, however, to emphasize the "hypothetical and provisional" nature of these explanations.[85]

Their hypothetical nature explained in part the textual work that diagrams could do. A plurality of *possible* diagrams could be deployed in order to elucidate some controverted question. Thus Bastian in 1898 employed no less than five such schemata in his attempt to express graphically the cerebral pathways that might account for the phenomenon of recovery from aphemia.[86] Each of these projected realities had its own plausibility; and the aphasiologist found work in weighing their relative merits.

The diagrams in question possessed an ambiguous ontological status. On the one hand, they were mere expository and heuristic devices. But, on the other hand, the circles and arrows of which they were composed

[83] Ibid., p. 491.
[84] Ibid., pp. 492–493.
[85] Ibid., pp. 493, 494.
[86] Bastian, *Treatise*, pp. 264–266.

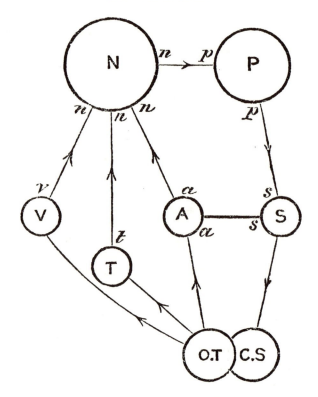

Figure 3.4. Diagram to illustrate hypothetical speech apparatus in the brain.
William Broadbent, "A Case of Peculiar Affection of Speech,
with Commentary" (1879)

were endowed with some relation, however tentative, to entities and processes supposedly contained in the "real" space of the configured brain. Thus, in an earlier publication, Bastian smoothly insinuated that "it may be assumed that the auditory and the visual word centres are situated, the one not far away from, and the other actually within some part of the cortex of the occipital lobe, and that they are connected together by a double set of commissural fibres."[87] The "it may be assumed" glided over the vertiginous chasm transversed in this process of translation. Conversely, the character of the convolutions and lobes of the cortex was also transformed by their verbal and graphic identification with the diagrammatic centers.

[87] H. Charlton Bastian, "On Different Kinds of Aphasia, With Special Reference to their Classification and Ultimate Pathology," *British Medical Journal* 2 (1887): 931–936, p. 933.

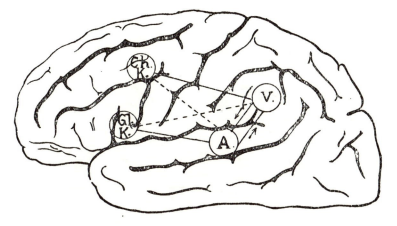

Figure 3.5. Superimposition of a diagram of the speech mechanism upon
a standard brain profile. H. Charlton Bastian, "Some Problems in
Connexion with Aphasia and other Speech Defects" (1897)

These ambiguities were highlighted by the practice that developed of
literally superimposing—or, to use Sigmund Freud's expression, *inscrib-
ing*—hypothetical diagrammatic features upon the standard brain profile
(see, for example, fig. 3.5).[88] The greater "reality" of the latter served to
enhance the credibility of the former. A schema could even, by means of
juxtaposition, be apparently *derived* from the more naturalistic form of
representation (fig. 3.6). When the external aspect of the head and such
details as a hand holding a pen were added to the design, the tentative
status of the diagram receded to be replaced by the implication that the
schema afforded an insight into the secret workings of the body (fig. 3.7).

These diagrams were also endowed with a predictive potential. From
them the symptoms accompanying any particular lesion could be read.
Henry Head, somewhat sardonically, recalled that:

> For eighteen years, at University College Hospital, Bastian had demonstrated
> to generations of students a man who had been seized with loss of speech in
> December 1877. On each occasion the famous diagram was drawn and we
> were told what commissural fibres were affected, and why the visual centre
> must be intact, although that for hearing was in a state of lowered vitality.[89]

---

[88] Sigmund Freud, *Zur Auffassung der Aphasien. Einer kritische Studie* (Leipzig: Franz
Deuticke, 1891), p. 9. Freud refers here, in particular, to Wernicke's diagram. He goes on
to note, however, that other diagrams, such as Lichtheim's, were too hypothetical to be thus
superimposed upon the real structures of the brain.

[89] Henry Head, *Aphasia and Kindred Disorders of Speech*, 2 vols. (Cambridge: Cambridge
University Press, 1926), vol. 1, pp. 56–57. Head went on to report that the findings of the
autopsy that terminated this case were not favorable to Bastian's predictions.

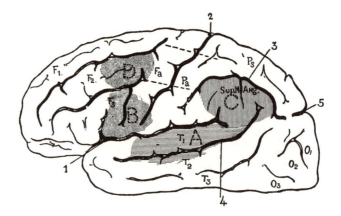

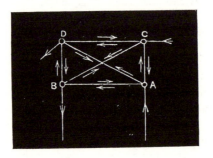

Figure 3.6. A schematic diagram purportedly derived from a more naturalistic representation. John Wyllie, *The Disorders of Speech* (1894)

This account illustrates the power that such diagrams exerted not only over cases and students, but also over the professor who demonstrated them. Clinical judgment was effectively deputed to these schemata.

The "clarity" and simplicity of these graphic devices could, moreover, serve to impose an explanatory order upon the obscurity and complexity of the aphasiological text. Dejerine, for instance, when discussing writing disorders, declared that "the following schema . . . allows us to respond to these different questions by at once explaining for us the mechanism in accordance with which reading and writing take place."[90] Such ascribed clarity made diagrams especially serviceable in pedagogical contexts: "Teachers of medicine could assume an easy dogmatism at the bedside

[90] Dejerine, "Contribution," p. 110.

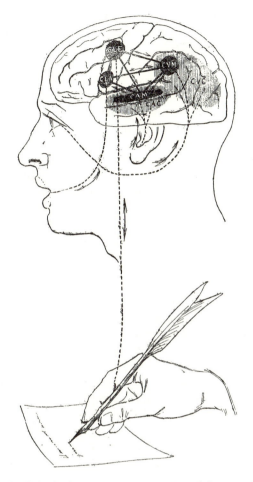

Figure 3.7. Embellished schematic representation of the speech mechanism.
Pierre Marie, "De l'aphasie" (1888)

and candidates for examination rejoiced in so perfect a clue to all their
difficulties."[91]

A diagram thus served to help lay down the law; to demonstrate the
order underlying apparent chaos.[92] Wernicke insisted that the generation
of all voluntary movements could be "reduced to [the] simple schema"

[91] Head, "Aphasia," p. 397.

[92] Henry Head was to condemn the species of rationalism that underlay this genre of
writing: "They failed to appreciate that the logical formulae of the intellect do not correspond absolutely to physical events and that the universe does not exist as an exercise for the
human mind. To them an explanation that appealed directly to reason must of necessity

he had provided. He maintained, moreover, that a particular pathway designated on another diagram "*adequately explains spontaneous movement in the mode of a reflex process.*"[93]

Such striving after law and order was one manifestation of an implicit scientism permeating the discourse of aphasia. Occasionally this bias became explicit. Ludwig Lichtheim declared that the method to be employed in aphasiology "does not differ from those used in the natural sciences. Starting from the observation of facts, it culminates in the explanation of these facts."[94] While this might be dismissed as a mere rhetorical gesture, the stylistic devices employed by Lichtheim and others in their attempts to constrain the phenomena of language within schematic bounds betrayed a yearning to approximate to idioms of more "exact" disciplines. Lichtheim's figures resemble those found in a text on geometry or mechanics (fig. 3.8). Wernicke supplemented such geometric conventions with the use of a quasi-algebraic notation.[95] In Adolf Kussmaul's *Die Störungen der Sprache* (1877) the (colored) diagram served in effect as a theorem from which certain corollaries could be derived.[96]

The question arises: What were these diagrams representations *of?* Certainly, they did not stand for concrete individuals or their lived experience of language in health or disease. The referent of these signs was a reality accessible only to the scientific gaze. Despite the obviously contrived nature of these representations, moreover, this was an objective field, not an artifact of scientific activity. Through the agency of these graphics, language and its disorders[97] were thus consigned to the realm of the other. The stylistic conventions as well as the modes of reasoning associated with the diagrammatic aspect of aphasiology witnessed a faith in the existence

---

correspond to the facts of observation; the form assumed by the manifestations of organic disease could be therefore confidently anticipated from study of a well considered diagram." Head, *Aphasia*, pp. 65–66.

[93] Wernicke, "Aphasia Symptom Complex," pp. 97–98 (10–12). In later writings by Wernicke the schema he had developed to explain sensory aphasia served as a template for conceptualizing a wide range of psychic disorders. See: Mario Horst Lanczik, Helmut Beckmann, and Gundolf Keil, "Wernicke," in German Berrios and Roy Porter (eds.), *A History of Clinical Psychiatry: The Origin and History of Psychiatric Disorders* (London, Athlone Press, 1995), pp. 303–6.

[94] Ludwig Lichtheim, "On Aphasia," *Brain* 7 (1885): 433–484, p. 433.

[95] See, for instance, Wernicke, "Aphasia Symptom Complex," p. 107 (28).

[96] Adolf Kussmaul, *Die Störungen des Sprache. Versuch einer Pathologie der Sprache* (Leipzig: F.C.W. Vogel, 1877), pp. 182–186. Cf. Head's remark that in Wernicke's work "the clinical forms of disordered speech are deduced from [the diagram] as from a figure in Euclid." Head, *Aphasia,* vol. 1, p. 62.

[97] The mere fact that these "processes" were deemed subject to graphic representation is, of course, itself an aspect of this strategy of visualizing in order to survey and dominate; "the human eye and ability to form concepts, are [supposed to be] the eternal witnesses of all things." Friedrich Nietzsche, *The Will to Power*, translated by Walter Kaufmann and R. J. Hollingdale (New York: Vintage Books, 1968), section 640.

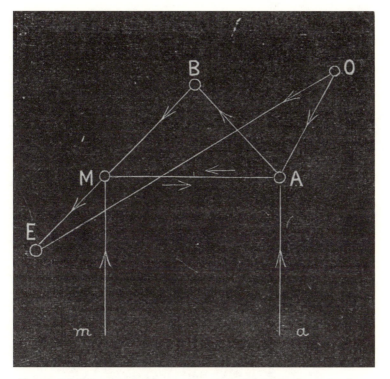

Figure 3.8. "Geometrical" representation of the speech mechanism.
Ludwig Lichtheim, "On Aphasia" (1885)

of a quasi-mathematical order underlying the phenomenal flux. Whatever the vagaries of any particular manifestation, the workings of the brain were represented as essentially lawful.[98] The task of aphasiology was to discern and depict this essence among the seeming disorder of the concrete instances of diseased speech presenting in the clinic. Textual manipulation of *the* brain aside, particular brains were subjected to various procedures designed to demonstrate their amenability to precise measurement and analysis (see figs. 3.9 and 3.10).

Diagrams, like the stereotyped cortical maps, moved freely about the aphasiological network and became a standard part of the kit with which workers in the field tackled their subject.[99] Bateman, for instance, invoked

[98] On mathematization as a more general trope in scientific representation see: Michael Lynch, "The Externalized Retina and Mathematization in the Visual Documentation of Objects in the Life Sciences," in M. Lynch and S. Woolgar, *Representation in Scientific Practice* (Cambridge, Mass.: MIT Press, 1990), pp. 169–170.

[99] Frederic Bateman reported that "One of the most interesting features of this meeting [of the British Association for the Advancement of Science in 1868] . . . was the discussion which followed the reading of papers on Aphasia by Dr. Hughlings Jackson, Mr Dunn, and

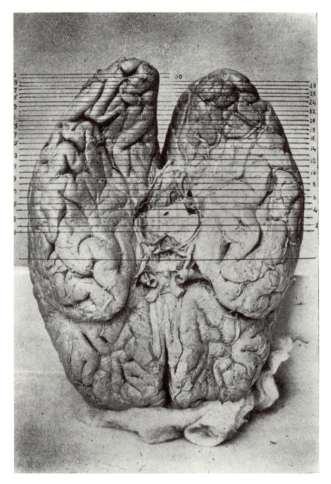

Figure 3.9. Photograph showing imposition of precise measures
on brain specimens. John Wyllie, *The Disorders of Speech* (1894)

Charcot's diagram, "and assuming for the moment that it contains, at
least, the germ of scientific truth, I will inquire what portion of the supposed speech-track was affected in the case I am now studying."[100] In an
1890 paper by Wernicke the diagram was ascribed a more authoritative
status. When confronted by a seemingly anomalous and difficult case he

---

M. Broca. The learned Parisian Professor, with great force and eloquence expounded before
a British audience, his own peculiar views as to the seat of speech, illustrating his remarks
by a coloured diagram, and a plaster cast. A most animated discussion ensued." Bateman,
"On Aphasia," p. 495.

[100] Bateman, *On Aphasia*, p. 141.

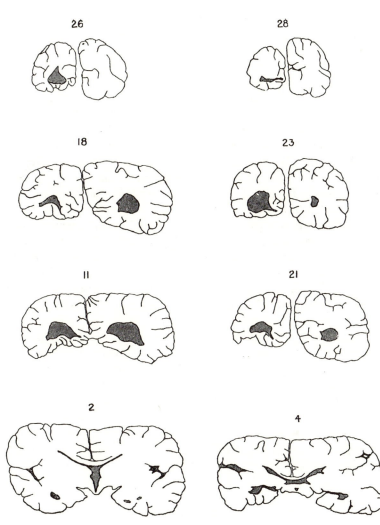

Figure 3.10. Cross-sections derived from previous figure.

concluded that "to solve the problem we must refer once more to the diagram we considered at the beginning of this discussion."[101] This schema was, in effect, to act as arbiter of the issue.

No diagram ever attained, however, the degree of general acceptance enjoyed by Gratiolet's classification of the cerebral convolutions. A form

[101] Carl Wernicke, "Aphasie und Geisteskrankheit," (1890) in *Gesammelte Aufsätze und kritische Referate zur Pathologie des Nervensystems* (Berlin: H. Kornfeld, 1893), p. 157.

of competition arose between diagrams with authors urging the superiority of one or other particular representation over its rivals. Sometimes discriminations seemed to be made on aesthetic grounds: Ross opined that although Charcot's diagram "is similar in its main outlines to Kussmaul's scheme, he has, with his usual illustrative power, rendered it more striking to the senses, and more easily comprehended at a glance than any hitherto advanced."[102] But more often the contest between diagrams revolved around issues of their relative adequacy as delineations of nature.

Bastian, in particular, stoutly maintained the superiority of his diagrams over rival designs. To this end, for instance, he juxtaposed Dejerine's schema for explaining word-blindness with one of his own.[103] While criticising Kussmaul's diagram, Lichtheim confessed that "I have some doubts as to whether [in one of his own schemata] the construction of the path of volitional writing is correct." He therefore offered an alternative design which might be more accurate: "Clinical observations," he declared, "are necessary to decide on this point also."[104] Lichtheim's avowed uncertainty thus generated work at both the textual level and at the bedside; as well as providing an opportunity to debate the relative merits of the two representations on offer, the obscurity of the point also demanded greater efforts from clinical investigators.

Lichtheim made obeisance to the fundamental status of clinical fact within the discourse of aphasia; but he also indicated the subordination of the accumulation of case histories within a system of higher-order objectives. Cases were significant in so far as they could contribute to the determination of controverted theoretical points. Patients were reduced to a species of dialectical cannon fodder; they were the occasions or opportunities for gaining additional insights, and, eventually, for the generation of new more accurate diagrams. The patient's body—and even "the brain" itself—were merely windows upon a purer, more perfect visual field.

Case Law

Diagrams formed one part of a panoply of devices available to aphasiology that served to define the patient's role within its emergent text. Those involved in the elaboration of this discourse were, for the most part, remarkably oblivious to the partialities of this mode of representing the alleged mechanisms of healthy and diseased language. A rare exception was John Wyllie who in 1894 conceded that "by localization and diagram-

---

[102] Ross, *On Aphasia*, p. 89.
[103] Bastian, "Some Problems," p. 1191.
[104] Lichtheim, "On Aphasia," pp. 440–443.

matic representation, we can, as yet, do no more than merely touch the fringe of the great question as to the nature of ideas, and their relation to speech. But it is something, even to touch the fringe of such a question."[105]

Within this text the "aphasic" arose in parallel with "the brain" as an abstract category to which concrete individuals more or less successfully approximated. The impulse to describe cases in terms of their exemplary value was evident even in the early history of the discourse. James Russell in 1864 commended a number of case histories to his readers on the grounds that they "afford a very striking illustration of the independence of the different functions of the nervous centres." One case was of special interest, "the patient presenting an excellent illustration" of a given form of speech defect.[106] At a later stage it became possible to speak of ideal patients who typified particular syndromes with only accidental reference to any particular historic individual. There was, in Charles Féré's formulation, such a thing as the "true aphasic."[107]

In his papers on "word-blindness" Dejerine illustrated how a clinical narrative could be structured by the need to relate the case in terms of a prior classificatory grid. The clinical history of one patient, he announced, "is made up of two stages." During the first stage "the patient presented the purest clinical picture imaginable of the second variety of word-blindness." During the second, much briefer, stage, the case had, however, been converted into one of the "first variety of word-blindness." Autopsy had revealed that to these two clinical stages there existed "two distinct anatomical lesions in the left hemisphere"; the later of which, "explains perfectly the symptoms observed in the last days of the patient's life."[108] The explanation was incomplete, however, until the cerebral mechanism that had been disrupted by these lesions was specified. Here a diagram came to Dejerine's aid: the facts were "easy to understand when one glances at the schema opposite."[109]

The value of patients was calculated in terms of their suitability for this kind of textual manipulation. Charcot displayed a classical sensibility when he congratulated his students on their good fortune in accumulating in his clinic several such "pathological cases of a truly remarkable purity. They will permit us to study the fundamental forms of the aphasic syndrome freed . . . from all admixture, from all complication, and consequently

---

[105] John Wyllie, *The Disorders of Speech* (Edinburgh: Oliver and Boyd, 1894), p. 279.

[106] Russell, "Hemiplegia," p. 408.

[107] Charles Féré, "Des troubles de l'usage des signes," *Revue philosophique* 17 (1884): 593–606, p. 598. For an account of the pathognomonic characteristics of the true aphasic see pp. 596–597.

[108] Dejerine, "Différentes variétés," pp. 83–84.

[109] Ibid., p. 85.

in conditions exceptionally favourable to physiological analysis."[110] Such individuals were of "interest" inasmuch as they approximated so closely to the aphasiologist's ideal.

Wernicke painted the "picture" of one such patient:

> *Apart from impairment in comprehension, the patient also presents aphasic symptoms in speech produced by absence of the unconscious monitoring of the imagery of the spoken word.* This lack is reflected in frequent word-confusion. The patient largely retains the ability to name objects, but this control tends to be very labile and is readily influenced by disposition and mood. There is no consistency of correct use of words. The patient does not possess a vocabulary of specific words which are always used correctly.[111]

Such a clinical picture corresponded to some characteristic lesion of the cortical machinery of language that was amenable to diagrammatic representation.

Wernicke conceded that these "pure clinical pictures" were usually obscured by the admixture of two or more of these symptom complexes in any given individual; the particularity of any given case was thus seen as ambient "noise" that had to be filtered out before useful information could be derived. He nonetheless insisted that "the typical pictures described, which themselves suffice to justify our formulation of a new clinical classification, actually do exist, (See the section on case-histories)."[112] Records of clinical facts were thus invoked to dispel any notion that Wernicke's "pictures" were merely imaginary constructs; their empirical referents were to be found in the case histories appended to his treatise.

The success of this validatory maneuver depended, however, upon suppressing the extent to which these narratives were themselves constructed in terms of the classification they were supposed to corroborate. Thus Case 3 was introduced as "a typical [*prägnanter*] case of conduction aphasia"[113]—a diagnosis that made sense only in the context of a preconceived notion of the mechanisms of language. Elsewhere Wernicke's exposition of his "clinical material" involved a direct quotation of the symbolic paraphenalia of his diagrams,[114] further vitiating the distinction between the schema and the empirical cases from which it was avowedly derived.

Wernicke's text exemplified a powerful impulse that characterized the entire discourse of aphasia. There was, if not a will to power, then a will to integrate the diversity of clinical presentation within a coherent and

---

[110] Charcot, "Des différentes formes," p. 441.

[111] Wernicke, "Aphasia Symptom Complex," p. 107 (pp. 23–24). Translation slightly modified.

[112] Ibid., p. 114 (32).

[113] Ibid., p. 126 (47).

[114] Ibid., pp. 135, 137–138 (59, 62).

comprehensive vision. "The theory of aphasia, here proposed," he maintained, "permits a consolidation of the different clinical pictures of the disorder. This diversity which formerly presented each new observer with fresh riddles to solve, will now no longer obtrude, in fact, they can now be calculated in accordance with the laws of combination."[115] All elements within the aphasiological text were obliged to submit to the imperative that they be law-abiding and calculable. Within the discourse of aphasia unity and coherence thus figured as a prime virtue while diversity was deemed a vice.

Whatever significance patients might have ascribed to their experience was strictly irrelevant. When a person heard voices he or she might ascribe them to spirits trying to communicate. Aphasiology revealed, however, that such "verbal hallucinations" were merely evidence of a determinate disorder in the cerebral speech centers. This diagnosis strictly circumscribed the range of permissible questions to be asked of the case. They could, in fact, be reduced to one: "What is the starting-point of the cerebral disturbances which produce these various hallucinations?"[116]

All cases in the archive—even those inscribed before the inception of aphasia proper—were subject to this regulation. In an especially telling move Lichtheim recalled Lordat's account of his alalia (see chapter 1) in order to make it conform to the laws he had outlined. The "celebrated case of Lordat," he insisted, "may be explained on the assumption of a simultaneous break in M B and A B."[117] Lordat's own depiction of his affliction as a lesion of the self was seemingly invisible to the aphasiologist's gaze, his case serving merely as further demonstration of the power of the diagram.

Conclusion

In his *De l'aphasie et de ses diverses formes* (1889) Désiré Bernard criticized a genre of medical writing that tried to find accounts of aphasia in earlier literature. The American neurologist William Hammond, for instance, found such cases in the Old Testament, the writings of classical authors like Thucydides and Pliny, as well as in various older medical texts.[118] Bernard's point was that it was fallacious to seek "aphasia" in documents that predated Broca's revolutionary contribution to the understanding of speech

[115] Ibid., p. 143 (69).
[116] Wyllie, *Disorders of Speech*, p. 204.
[117] Lichtheim, "On Aphasia," p. 465.
[118] William A. Hammond, *A Treatise on the Diseases of the Nervous System* (New York: D. Appleton, 1886), pp. 184–185.

loss. It was only after Broca had described the condition that it became possible for aphasia to possess a textual existence. If one were to seek a true account of the condition in imaginative literature, it was necessary to look to writing in the modern, post-1861 period. Bernard cited, in particular, "M. Émile Zola who, as early as 1867, depicted an aphasic in the moving pages of *Thérèse Raquin*, with a perfect understanding of what he wrote."[119]

The "aphasic" in question was Madame Raquin, mother-in-law to Thérèse and her second husband Laurent. The couple are tormented by the memory of Madame Raquin's son who, unbeknown to her, they murdered. Madame Raquin's presence in the household gives some comfort to the guilty pair: "All the while the two murderers were sitting, silent and still, at her side, apparently listening devoutly to what she was saying; in reality, however, they made no effort to follow the poor old woman's ramblings, but were just glad of this quiet flow of words, which prevented them from hearing their own clamorous thoughts."[120]

However, one evening as Madame Raquin was engaged in such a monologue, "she stopped in mid-sentence. . . . When she tried to scream, and call for help, she could only come out with rasping noises. Her tongue had turned to stone, her hands and feet had gone stiff. She had been struck dumb and immobilized." This sudden transformation appalled Thérèse and Laurent:

> they realized that what they had in front of them was now no more than a body half alive, which could see and hear them, but not speak. This attack plunged them into despair, not because they were concerned at the paralysed woman's sufferings, but out of self-pity, because they would have to live from now on with only each other for company.[121]

The effect of this calamity upon these two was, however, as nothing compared to the predicament of Madame Raquin herself. She had become

---

[119] Désiré Bernard, *De l'aphasie et de ses diverses formes* (Paris: Lecrosnier and Babé, 1886), p. 7. For a somewhat superficial discussion of the place of the medical in Zola's novels see: Garabed Eknoyan and Byron A. Eknoyan, "Medicine and the Case of Émile Zola," in Bruce Clarke and Wendell Aycock, *The Body and the Text: Comparative Essays in Literature and Medicine* (Lubbock: Texas Tech University Press, 1990), pp. 103–114. The case of aphasia in *Thérèse Raquin* does not figure in the authors' list of "Diseases in Zola's Writings." For a far more insightful appreciation of the place of the medical in Zola's work see: Lawrence Rothfield, *Vital Signs: Medical Realism in Nineteenth-Century Fiction* (Princeton: Princeton University Press, 1992), pp. 6–8, 127–129. Rothfield, however, argues that the model of experimental medicine, rather than the merely clinical gaze, was predominant in Zola's later work.

[120] Émile Zola, *Thérèse Raquin*, trans. Andrew Rothwell, (Oxford: Oxford University Press), p. 143.

[121] Ibid., p. 155.

a "walled-in intelligence, still alive but buried deep within a dead body. . . . Her mind was akin to one of those people who are accidentally buried alive and who wake up in the darkness of the earth . . . ; they struggle and shout, and others walk around on top of them without hearing their dreadful lamentations." As Laurent, with uncharacteristic insight, remarked, "There must be some cruel drama going on deep down in that useless body of hers."[122]

The drama becomes yet more cruel when Madame Raquin accidentally learns about the murder of her son. Because of her bodily condition she is unable to communicate this knowledge and so bring the criminals to justice. Recognizing that she had no means to exact retribution, "she resigned herself to silence and immobility, and great tears fell slowly from her eyes. Nothing could be more heart-rending than this still, wordless grief of hers."[123]

Zola's account of aphasia thus concentrates upon the devastating effects of the condition for the status of the self, both as an actor in the social world, and in her own subjective interiority. Once struck dumb Madame Raquin ceases to possess even the feeble social presence she had once enjoyed; she becomes a mere "it" to be contemplated with pity and horror by others. Moreover, in her own consciousness her selfhood assumes a monstrous aspect: she is a mind with no control over her body, which, far from being her instrument, is now her prison. Above all, she can no longer have any influence on the world around her. The pathos of her situation is heightened by the fact that she now possesses vital information which she is incapable of imparting to others.

Bernard's compliments on the medical accuracy of Zola's narrative notwithstanding, the discourse of aphasia was only marginally, when at all, concerned with such issues. Its chief preoccupation was with the classification of a pathology of which the individual was accidentally the seat. What mattered was to find a "pure" and "simple" case that would provide a "veritable schema" of a particular form of aphasia.[124]

Occasionally, however, authors did indicate that an awareness of the *kind* of individual that served as host to a particular lesion might be of some heuristic significance. Starr remarked that "The scholar who constantly studies and the laborer who reads only the street-signs will be very differently effected [*sic*] by a lesion producing a loss of the visual memories. These distinctions of mental power therefore cannot be disregarded in the study of a disease which touches the physical basis of mind."[125] Such

---

[122] Ibid., pp. 158–159.

[123] Ibid., p. 162.

[124] See the remarks in: Gilbert Ballet, *Le langage intérieur et les formes diverses de l'aphasie* (Paris: Félix Alcan, 1886), pp. 82–83, 104.

[125] Starr, "Aphasia," p. 332.

nuances were of special relevance to the proper therapy to be applied in a given case (see chapter 7).

Some aphasiological texts even registered, in much the same way as had Zola, the pathos of a self thus afflicted. Trousseau noted of one patient at the Hôtel-Dieu:

> his expression indicates intelligence, but it is impossible for him to reply to any of our questions. . . . He hears well fixing his eyes on us when we question him; his gestures, his eyes show that he understands what we say, it seems that thoughts fill his brain, but he is unable to express them by speech.

But it is still the "local modifications" that have occurred in the substance of this brain that are Trousseau's principal concern.[126]

The patient that invoked these observations from Trousseau was a "young working-man." But, as Starr's remarks indicate, the individuality of persons of higher social status was thought more likely to impinge upon the expression of their pathology. The fact that a particular patient had "received quite a good education, since he attended a seminary and had aimed to be a priest," meant that it "will be easier for us to study the degradations of the intelligence and to appreciate all its manifestations."[127] This was a hospital patient. When, however, the case was one encountered in private practice then the individuality of the patient merited a more detailed attention.

When narrating the case of the wealthy "M. X." whom he had been summoned to attend in the spring of 1863, Trousseau recorded that

> I found a man of very agreeable appearance, very neat, even elegant. . . . His face is intelligent, kindly, smiling. He gets up when I arrive and indicates the pleasure he feels in seeing me by means of gesture and above all by the expression of his features. However, he does not speak and merely babbles entirely unintelligble words.[128]

This account is in certain respects reminiscent of aspects of Lordat's case histories (see chapter 1), an impression strengthened in what follows.

Trousseau also noted that at dinner M. X. ate "very properly and with infinitely more reserve than the majority of paralytics." He was, moreover, courteous to his hosts, seeking by means of gesture to participate in the table talk. He even indicated which of the wines on offer was the finest. The emphasis is therefore upon the extent to which M. X.'s status as a man of culture and feeling has survived his affliction. Only when Trousseau subsequently tested his reading abilities is there any hint of

---

[126] Trousseau, *Clinique médicale*, pp. 571–572.
[127] Ibid., p. 581.
[128] Ibid., p. 584.

the subjective consequences of the injury he has suffered: "He fixed the title of the book with his eyes for some time; but after several seconds, he threw the book away with an ill humour that testified to his impotence." The patient had retained, however, his skill as a card player. More importantly, he remained competent to understand the management of his financial affairs.[129]

When dealing with persons of property this last was a point of some significance. In this context, the question of the continued integrity of the self became intertwined with that of the survival of the legal and economic subject. Trousseau took care to note of one lady, whose vocabulary was restricted to the phrase *Sacré nom de Dieu*, that she was still a competent actor in the marketplace.[130] An important appendix to the discourse of aphasia dealt with the forensic question of determining the capacity of individuals who no longer had full command of the faculty of language to manage their own affairs.[131] The question tended to arise, however, only when the patient was a man or woman of property.

Aphasiology was capable of adopting novelistic devices to depict the phenomenology of the condition when the self in question seemed to warrant such treatment. Writing of a multilingual merchant who had possessed an extraordinary *mémoire visuelle*, Charcot resorted to the device of free indirect speech to represent the impact of an aphasic attack upon this individual. After a period of unusually intense business worries,

> M. X. was struck abruptly with a profound change in himself. . . . [F]rom that time a violent contrast arose between his former and his new state. So much did the things around him seem new and strange that M. X. felt himself for a moment menaced with madness. He had become nervous and irritable. In all events, his visual memory of forms and colours had entirely vanished, as he quickly recognized, and this realization reassured him about his mental state. He later learned that he could, by other means, by invoking different forms of memory, competently continue to direct his commercial affairs.[132]

Nonetheless, whenever M. X. entered his hometown, "it seemed to him that he was entering a place unknown to him."[133]

Charcot was willing to acknowledge an intellectual parity between himself and this patient—who had already himself arrived at most of the same conclusions as his doctor about the nature of his case. Charcot even concluded the case history with a note composed at his request by M. X.

---

[129] Ibid., pp. 584–585.

[130] Ibid., p. 616.

[131] See Bateman, *On Aphasia*, chapter X on the jurisprudence of aphasia.

[132] J.-M. Charcot, *Leçons sur les maladies du système nerveux faites à la Salpêtrière* (Paris: A. Delahaye and E. Lecrosnie, 1887), p. 179.

[133] Ibid., p. 180.

himself in which the patient expatiated further upon "the complete change that has taken place in my existence" and the consequent alteration of his "character."[134] Charcot demonstrated his respect for M. X.'s words by declining to engage in any extensive editorialization of this letter; the patient was allowed to speak for himself.[135]

No such respect was accorded, however, to the great majority of the individuals who contributed their afflictions, and often their bodies also, to the erection of the edifice of aphasiology. Their speech, in so far as it persisted, was recorded merely because it was symptomatic of underlying pathology rather than significant in itself. The true referent of their words was a lesion of the brain, not a deformed self. A speechless individual entering a late nineteenth-century hospital was confronted with an immense *épaisseur* of writing which absorbed and redefined him or her according to its own discursive logic and imperatives.[136] The speechless patient became the aphasic, and was assigned to the realm of nature.

[134] Ibid., p. 184.
[135] Ibid., p. 186.
[136] On Foucault's concept of discursive density see: Goldstein, "Foucault among the Sociologists," p. 188.

FOUR

JOHN HUGHLINGS JACKSON AND
THE PREDICAMENT OF THE
"SPEECHLESS MAN"

What therefore is truth? A mobile army of metaphors,
metonymies, anthropomorphisms: in short a sum of
human relations.
*(Friedrich Nietzsche, "Of Truth and Falsity
in their Ultramoral Sense")*

"The first great advance of the human race," said the
Professor, "was when, by the development of their left frontal
convolutions, they developed the power of speech. Their
second advance was when they learned to control that power.
Woman has not yet attained the second stage."
(Arthur Conan Doyle, "A Physiologist's Wife")

I N 1915 the British neurologist Henry Head reviewed the development of aphasiology from the 1860s to the 1890s. His judgment was
damning. "It is generally conceded," he declared, "that the views on
aphasia and analogous disturbances of speech found in the text-books of
to-day are of little help in understanding an actual case of disease." The
fault—"an old failing in medical history"—lay in an excessive desire for
clarity and precision at the expense of attention to the nuances—the sheer
facticity—of any particular case; as a result of this impulse,

> Each patient with a speech defect of cerebral origin is stretched on the pro-
> crustean bed of some theoretical scheme: something is lopped away at one
> part, something added at another, until the phenomena are said to corre-
> spond to some diagrammatic conception, which never has and never could
> have existed. And yet neurologists continue to cling to these schemes, modi-
> fying them to suit each case, conscious that they do not correspond in any
> way to the facts they are supposed to explain.[1]

---

[1] Henry Head, "Hughlings Jackson on Aphasia and Kindred Affections of Speech," *Brain*
38 (1915): 1–27, pp. 1–2.

Head had, in effect, identified in the practice of previous aphasiologists traits that Nietzsche regarded as a universal tendency: "The power of the spirit to appropriate what is foreign to it is revealed in a strong inclination to assimilate the new to the old, to simplify the complex, to overlook or repel what is wholly contradictory." Conversely, "the same will is served by an apparently antithetical drive of the spirit, a sudden decision for ignorance, for arbitrary shutting-out, . . . an acceptance and approval of ignorance."[2]

To those working within a discourse the validity of such biases and exclusions appeared self-evident—*natural* rather than arbitrary. Indeed, they only became visible at the point when the legitimacy of a way of life began to be challenged; then their artifice becomes obvious and even offensive. A new sensibility has arisen under which the natural assumptions of others become outrageous to the texture of reality. The place of Head's critique of classical aphasiology in the so-called holist movement in neurology at the turn of the twentieth century will be considered in the following chapter.[3] Here I am concerned with the honorable exception Head identified to the generally deplorable state of previous aphasia studies.

In Head's view, John Hughlings Jackson (1835–1911)[4] "was one of the most remarkable pioneers in the field of defects of speech caused by cerebral disease." Jackson published a large number of articles on the subject between 1864 and 1893, although he never collected his opinions into a monograph. He also used his position at the National Hospital for Nervous Diseases at Queen's Square in London as a platform from which to instruct generations of medical men in his views on the nature of these conditions. Despite these efforts, "even amongst the younger men [Jackson's] aphoristic dicta fell upon deaf ears."[5]

Head adduced four reasons for the neglect Jackson had suffered in his own lifetime. The first was a matter of character: Jackson's private virtues militated against the proper dissemination of his ideas. He was "a man of such profound personal modesty that he laid little value on the publication of his views." Second there was the peculiarity of the language in which

---

[2] Friedrich Nietzsche, *Beyond Good and Evil: Prelude to a Philosophy of the Future*, translated R. J. Hollingdale (London: Penguin, 1990), pp. 160–161.

[3] On this phenomenon see Anne Harrington, " 'A Feeling for the 'Whole': The Holistic Reaction in Neurology from the *Fin de Siècle* to the Interwar Years," in Mikulas Teich and Roy Porter (eds.), *Fin de Siècle and its Legacy* (Cambridge: Cambridge University Press, 1990), pp. 254–277; idem, *Reenchanted Science: Holism in German Culture from Wilhelm II to Hitler* (Princeton: Princeton University Press, 1996).

[4] For biographical information see: Samuel H. Greenblatt, "The Major Influences on the Early Life and Work of John Hughlings Jackson," *Bulletin of the History of Medicine* 39 (1965): 346–376.

[5] Head, "Hughlings Jackson," p. 2.

Jackson expressed his dicta; his style was, Head conceded, "peculiarly difficult to read." This apparent fault was, however, properly conceived as further proof of Jackson's intellectual integrity. The "bristling difficulties of Hughlings Jackson's papers" were to be more esteemed than the "fluent facility of his contemporaries."[6] The tortuous nature of Jackson's language reflected his unremitting struggle with the intractability of the phenomena he strove to describe.

A third difficulty lay in Jackson's resort to terminology derived from the works of the philosopher Herbert Spencer to provide a theoretical framework for his observations. These usages had tended "to alienate psychologists, blinding them to the truths underlying this somewhat uncouth nomenclature."[7] The "truths" embodied in Jackson's insights were therefore somehow independent of the concepts through which they were articulated; they might be translated into a more acceptable jargon—although Head declined to undertake this task.

Head's final explanation for Jackson's neglect was virtually redundant: "the nature of the ideas he propounded was foreign to the current views of the day." His were the utterances of a disregarded prophet. Jackson was credited with the wisdom to have appreciated this fact himself. Head attributed to him the aphorism that: "it generally takes a truth twenty-five years to become known in medicine."

Head thus portrayed Jackson as a saint to science—as one whose devotion to truth overrode any vulgar desire for public recognition, one who had the humility to put the facts before reason, and to privilege difficulty above clarity. Such virtue did, however, have its eventual reward. "Each generation of house physicians and clinical clerks at the National Hospital," Head declared, "passed out impressed by the beauty of his character and his simple-hearted sincerity. Some carried away with them one or more of his broad generalizations to bear fruit in their subsequent work."[8] The moral characteristics and the scientific doctrines of the man are thus presented as inseparable.

But such direct personal influence was necessarily limited in its scope. If Jackson's influence was to extend beyond the few who had been privileged to imbibe his manna by direct personal contact, it had to be through the agency of his writings. And it was to this end that Head reprinted a collection of Jackson's articles on aphasia and affections of speech in the neurological journal *Brain*.

What made Jackson's writings on aphasia distinctive was the respect he gave to the *facts* of the cases he described. Deference to fact was, of course,

---

[6] Ibid., pp. 2–3.
[7] Ibid., p. 3.
[8] Ibid.

commonplace; but Head maintained that for most of Jackson's contemporaries such reverence was mere lip service. They were too intent on forcing the facts into some preconceived schema, preferably embodied in diagrammatic form. In contrast,

> Jackson's attitude was strictly phenomenal. He never deduced his observations from his hypothesis, but any hypothesis he enunciated sprang, as it were, ready made from some clinical fact. . . . He stood like an observer on a bridge formulating the extent of the flood from matter carried down by the stream.[9]

Above all, Jackson was unique in his recognition that these "phenomena are primarily psychical and only in the second place susceptible of physiological or anatomical explanation."[10]

Head's was among the first of many icons of John Hughlings Jackson to be constructed. While sharing certain general features in common— they all tend to agree that Jackson's work represents a significant moment in the emergence of modern neurology—these have tended to diverge in matters of detail and emphasis. Different, and on occasions incompatible, achievments have been ascribed to the hero. Where these representations agree is in the view that Jackson effected a revolution in the language of neurology; indeed, some claim that his work provided the conditions for authentic neurological discourse.[11]

I do not propose to provide a survey of the various images of John Hughlings Jackson that have circulated during the twentieth century. Instead this chapter takes as its starting point Head's characterization of what was distinctive about Jackson's way of writing about affections of language with a cerebral origin. It analyzes in particular Jackson's account of the peculiarly "psychic" aspect of these phenomena in order to estimate the adequacy of Head's image of Jackson as a detached observer of the flow of clinical facts. It will argue that these facts have no existence independent of the discourse in which they are embedded. This linguistic practice was, moreover, imbued with some of the fundamental values and dichotomies of nineteenth-century culture.

Jackson's Way of Writing

Certain aspects of Jackson's work are entirely representative of the genre of medical writing about language and the brain that developed after 1861

---

[9] Ibid., p. 6.

[10] Ibid., p. 4

[11] See, for example, H. Tristram Engelhardt, "John Hughlings Jackson and the Mind-Body Relation," *Bulletin of the History of Medicine* 49 (1975): 137–151, pp. 143–144.

(chapter 2). Indeed, his earliest contributions read like typical examples of archive building: "I bring forward in this paper," began an 1864 piece, "thirty-four cases of hemiplegia, in all of which loss of speech, in a greater or less degree, was present."[12]

At all stages in his literary career, moreover, he displayed the scientism inherent in the aphasiological project. Indeed, Jackson incorporated the goals of scientific medicine into his presentation of self. "For some years," he avowed in 1873, "I have studied cases of disease of the brain, not only for direct, but for anatomical and physiological purposes." He reiterated the conventional view that affections of the nervous system should be regarded "as the results of experiments made by disease on particular parts of the nervous system of man." Indeed, the negative effects of "destroying" lesions and the positive results of "discharging" lesions precisely paralleled the operations of the physiologist upon an experimental subject.[13]

Although he was thus faithful to some of the most basic goals of aphasiology, from an early stage in his career Jackson's texts came to manifest less typical tendencies. He began, in particular, to show a more critical interest in the categories within which aphasiology framed and addressed its questions than any of his contemporaries, with the possible exception of Henry Maudsley. Jackson was especially scathing about the casual way in which his colleagues combined terms from what were for him incompatible spheres of discourse:

> Among those who believe that their method of studying those nervous diseases in which there are mental symptoms is anatomical or physiological, there are some whose method is neither, but practically psychological only. For they speak as if at some place in the higher parts of the nervous system we abruptly cease to have to do with impressions and movements, and begin all at once to have to do with mental states. There are motor centres, and above these centres for ideas, for memory, volition, etc., which "play on" the motor centres. . . . Even admitting the truth of each of these statements, taken separately, the mildest criticism on the coupling of them is, that in one case psychological language is used, and in the other anatomico-physiological language.[14]

[12] John Hughlings Jackson, "Loss of Speech: Its Association with Valvular Disease of the Heart and with Hemiplegia on the Right Side.—Defects of Smell.—Defects of Speech in Chorea.—Arterial Lesions in Epilepsy [1864]," in "Reprint of Some of Dr. Hughlings Jackson's Papers on Affections of Speech," *Brain* (1915): 28–42, p. 28.

[13] John Hughlings Jackson, "On the Anatomical and Physiological Localization of Movements in the Brain [1873]," in "Reprint," 75–79, p. 75.

[14] John Hughlings Jackson, "Notes on the Physiology and Pathology of Language," in "Reprint," 48–58, p. 48. See also Jackson, "Remarks on Evolution and Dissolution of the Nervous System," *Journal of Mental Science* 33 (1888): 25–48, p. 41.

By drawing attention to the metaphorical character of the relationship conventionally posited between the "psychic" and the motor nervous centers, Jackson attempted to cast doubt on the veridical status of this account of the organization of the brain: such devices were evidence of linguistic *artifice* rather than truthful accounts of nature. Sigmund Freud was to adopt a similar strategy in his own critique of classical aphasiology (see chapter 6). Jackson himself laid claim to a linguistic practice in which the subjective and objective aspects of nervous disorders were kept rigorously apart at an analytic level, but which at the same time acknowledged the intermingling of mental and physical symptoms in the clinic.

As well as such theoretical recommendations, Jackson purported to provide an example of how clinical description might be purged of tendentious elements in order to produce a pure description of what was encountered at the patient's bedside. It was, for example, "certainly . . . better to record the fact that the patient does not put out his tongue when told, than the inference that it is paralysed. . . . Here, again, we shall do no harm to clinical medicine if we simply record all the facts."[15] In reports of his own clinical practice Jackson on occasion reinforced these calls for an unassuming form of description with shows of modesty that conceded the possibility of personal error.[16] Paradoxically, however, such autobiographical reminiscence also had the effect of rendering Jackson a highly visible character in his text.

The first person pronoun in fact figures prominently in Jackson's writing; but this sign does not have a constant referent.[17] The "I" is sometimes, as we have seen, the historical John Hughlings Jackson, who pursued physiological as well as clinical research and who sometimes agonized over the accuracy of his case notes. This was, moreover, an embodied ego—inasmuch, at least, as he possessed a little finger for a certain patient to grasp.[18]

But other usages of the pronoun are more problematic. The contrast is on occasion apparent within the same passage:

When I am to think of a place I have once visited, I "see" faintly some part of it which has struck me most, e.g., of Petersfield, the market place; or for a certain village, the Green, where there are railings under an elm tree. Such

---

[15] Jackson, "Loss of Speech," p. 37.

[16] Jackson, "Notes . . . Language," p. 50. Protestation of modesty was a well-established device for claiming scientific credibility; see: Steven Shapin and Simon Schaffer, *Leviathan and the Air-Pump: Hobbes, Boyle, and the Experimental Life* (Princeton: Princeton University Press, 1985), pp. 65–69.

[17] See: Dalia Judovitz, *Subjectivity and Representation in Descartes: The Origins of Modernity* (Cambridge: Cambridge University Press, 1988), p. 4.

[18] Jackson, "Notes . . . Language," p. 50.

fragments stand to me, I conceive, as counters in ordinary thought for the whole place. If I am made to think of a place I have never seen, but have read of, I have still some visions of maps or of names on maps.[19]

Here the "I" in some instances still refers to an empirical self with particular experiences and memories of specific places. But by the final sentence, if not before, it has modulated into a transcendent subject of thought untrammeled by any historical particularity. This "I" is no longer a representation of John Hughlings Jackson but the sign of every rational man. He is the familiar protagonist—simultaneously both subject and object—of metaphysical writing since the time of Descartes.[20] It is this grammatical subject that predominates in the "psychological" analysis contained in Jackson's texts.

When Head commended Jackson for his emphasis upon the "psychic" side of aphasic disorders, he implied that this type of analysis dealt with a pristine, unmediated reality. An attention to inner experience was, in particular, a needful antidote to the artificial schemata and diagrams of those who sought to understand these morbid events as processes occuring in some imaginary outer space. As part of his critique of the basic axioms of Western philosophy, however, Nietzsche had challenged such assumptions: he denied, in particular, the erroneous starting point that there existed " 'facts of consciousness'—and no phenomenalism in introspection."[21]

Nietzsche extended his relativistic understanding of representations of external reality to the data of introspection. "Thinking," he declared, "as epistemologists conceive it, simply does not occur: it is a quite arbitrary fiction, arrived at by selecting one element from the process and eliminating all the rest, an artificial arrangment for the purpose of intelligibility."[22] The structuring of inner reality was "arbitrary" inasmuch as the order discerned there was not necessary or given by the facts of introspection themselves; but the process of selection and arrangement was not random or left to individual whim. Nietzsche insisted that "a correlation exists

---

[19] Jackson, "Notes on the Physiology and Pathology of the Nervous System [1868]," in "Reprint," 65–71, p. 70.

[20] See: James A. Winders, *Gender, Theory, and the Canon* (Madison: University of Wisconsin Press, 1991), chapter 2.

[21] Friedrich Nietzsche, *The Will to Power*, translated by Walter Kaufmann and R. J. Hollingdale (New York: Vintage Books, 1968), section 475.

[22] Ibid., section 477. The point can perhaps be emphasized by insisting upon the *textual* character of all representations of the psyche; whatever metaphor may be chosen to delineate psychical reality, Derrida's remark on Freud's machine/writing model of memory applies: "there is no domain of the psychic without text." "Freud and the Scene of Writing," in *Writing and Difference*, trans. Alan Bass (London: Routledge, 1993), pp. 196–231, on p. 199.

between degrees of value and degrees of reality (so that the supreme values also possess the supreme reality)." In other words, "Our values are interpreted *into* things."[23] The metaphysical order was necessarily a moral order.

The Duality of Mind

A defining characteristic of the metaphysical subject was its disembodied status; the "mind" could allegedly know itself without reference to the body.[24] Corporeal aspects of being were relegated to the status of the incidental. Given that Jackson was a medical writer whose avowed primary interest was in diseases of the body, this disembodiment might seem to constitute a fundamental difficulty.

In fact, the subject in his writing does appear to *have* a body—although it is not itself corporeal. When describing how it is possible for the subject to have a notion of a general category such as "horse," Jackson writes:

> There have long been permanent modifications of my brain which make it possible for another person at any time to *compel me* to have in my consciousness, at least momentarily, unless I am strongly preoccupied, *some* kind of notion of horse. He excites certain changes in the "grooves" of those permanent modifications of my brain which are always with me, part of me.[25]

"I" therefore possesses a brain which is integral to its capacities—its unique modifications are a "part of me."

The corporeality with which the subject is equipped (if not encumbered) is not, however, the familiar body of everyday discourse. It is, on the contrary, constructed from the terms of esoteric medical theory. This refined corporeality is what the subject possesses and on which it is to some degree dependent for its character and operations. The vulgar body remains elusive if not invisible. When he came to specify the morphology and dynamics of the mind/brain couplet at the center of his psychology, Jackson resorted to a number of basic dichotomies. Jackson was, in partic-

---

[23] Ibid., sections 583, 590.

[24] Cf. Derrida's comments on Husserl's phenomenology, which he regards as caught up in the tradition of metaphysics: "everything that escapes the pure spiritual intention, the pure animation by *Geist*, that is, the will, is excluded from meaning . . . and thus from expression. What is excluded is, for example, facial expressions, gestures, the whole of the body and the mundane register, in a word, the whole of the visible and spatial as such." *Speech and Phenomena and Other Essays on Husserl's Theory of Signs* (Evanston: Northwestern University Press, 1973), p. 35.

[25] Jackson, "Notes . . . Nervous System," p. 69.

ular, "to urge the *doubleness* of mental processes";[26] a corresponding duplex form was apparent in the brain.

A recent study of the history of the concept of the duality of cerebral action has declared that "Nineteenth-century thought on brain duality and functional asymmetry reached its climax in the person of John Hughlings Jackson."[27] It would be more accurate to say that the notion of the duality of mental and *therefore* cerebral operation formed a central trope in Jackson's writings. As Harrington implies, this was no personal idiosyncracy, but expressive of a disseminated cultural preoccupation with division and distinction in the realm of human action. His notion of the nature of cerebrally determined affections of language was shaped by this tendency; indeed, Jackson insisted that "the phenomena of cases of aphasia most clearly illustrate the nature of the duality of mental operations."[28]

One fundamental diremption that Jackson reproduced in his account of the workings of the mind/brain was that between active and passive, the voluntary and the automatic. "It seems plain," Jackson affirmed, "that there is, at least often—always, I imagine—involuntary prior to voluntary revival of perceptions." For example,

> When I hear a certain creaking noise, I "see," in spite of myself, a certain room. I should have so *suffered* any time in the last twenty years, and may for the next twenty. Here a simple sensation rouses a perception. . . . In short, the sensation first acts upon me as it finds me, unawares. I am suddenly its victim, for it brings the room before me in spite of me. On the other hand, it was possible for the "I" to " 'will' to dwell on the perception which has been obtruded on me, and for this there would, I presume, be required a *voluntary* revival of the perception."[29]

Corresponding to this psychic duality was a similarly differentiated concept of brain function. There was a voluntary, or "leading," side to the brain and an involuntary, or "automatic," side. The phenomena of aphasia were to be understood in these terms:

> the fundamental defect in loss of speech from disease in one hemisphere is inability to reproduce words voluntarily, because the leading motor part of one (the left) side of the brain is damaged. Involuntary reproduction (understanding words) remains possible, because the automatic side (right) is intact.

[26] Ibid., p. 65.
[27] Anne Harrington, *Medicine, Mind, and the Double Brain: A Study in Nineteenth-Century Thought* (Princeton: Princeton University Press, 1987), p. 206.
[28] John Hughlings Jackson, "On the Anatomical and Physiological Localisation of Movements in the Brain [1875]," in James Taylor (ed.), *Selected Writings of John Hughlings Jackson*, 2 vols. (London: Hodder and Stoughton, 1931), vol. 1, p. 38.
[29] Jackson, "Notes . . . Nervous System," p. 68.

Thus, reduced to its simplest form, loss of speech corresponds to hemiplegia, in which form of palsy the voluntary movements are lost, the involuntary preserved.[30]

The healthy subject therefore possessed a power to "propositionize" as well as the capacity to receive propositions. In the former exercise he or she was an active agent; in the latter the "victim" of another speaker. Separate nervous arrangements were posited for each of these actions and a hierarchy established between the two sides of the brain; the left was the "leading," because voluntary, hemisphere. Aphasia (using the term generically) was, thus conceived, essentially a defect of voluntary control.

Jackson's concept of the mechanisms of language was, to take Head's view, assembled from assiduous observations made from his metaphorical bridge of the psychological, clinical, and pathological phenomena. No "hypothesis" intruded into the process. Head's metaphor implied, however, that Jackson possessed some superior vantage point from which to observe the flow of facts: he was not immersed in that stream; he was above it. If Jackson was not standing on some structure derived from hypothesis, of what *was* his bridge composed?

Head's account of Jackson's cognitive processes is neither more nor less fanciful than any other. What can be said with some certainty, however, is that the textual embodiment of the results of these labors reveals not only a series of facts, but also a system of values. Indeed, the values make the facts what they are. By seeking to identify these values we may gain some insight into the materials that went into the construction of Jackson's cognitive "bridge."

Word, Will, and Power

Jackson's "debt" to the writings of Herbert Spencer has often been noted[31]—not least by Jackson himself. This debt is ususally conceived as a matter of theoretical borrowing; Jackson is, in particular, deemed to have owed his notion of the evolution and dissolution of nervous function to

---

[30] Jackson, "Abstract of the Gulstonian Lectures on Certain Points in the Study and Classification of Diseases of the Nervous System [1869]," in "Reprint," 72–74, p. 73.

[31] For instance, Samuel H. Greenblatt, "Hughlings Jackson's First Encounter with the Work of Paul Broca: The Physiological and Philosophical Background," *Bulletin of the History of Medicine* 44 (1970): 555–570, p. 568; idem, "The Development of Hughlings Jackson's Approach to Diseases of the Nervous System 1863–1866: Unilateral Seizures, Hemiplegia and Aphasia," *Bull. Hist. Med.* 51 (1977): 412–430, p. 427. For a fuller discussion of the relations between Spencer and Jackson see: C. U. M. Smith, "Evolution and the Problem of Mind: Part I. Herbert Spencer," *Journal of the History of Biology* 15 (1982): 55–88; "Part II. John Hughlings Jackson," ibid., 241–62.

this source.[32] Less comment has been made on Jackson's use of the Spencerian notion of "the survival of the fittest" in his characterization of psychic and nervous processes.

On this view, Spencer figures as a biological theorist who supplied Jackson with a number of useful conceptual tools that proved applicable to his own special concerns. Such borrowing within science is commonplace and requires no particular explication or comment. But this notion of the influence of one author upon another, while necessary and undeniable, is inadequate fully to characterize the community between Spencer's and Jackson's texts.

Spencer was far more than a biological author narrowly conceived; he aspired to create a synthetic philosophy that would encompass all aspects of nature, man, and society.[33] He maintained, in particular, that evolution was an universal principle for understanding the whole of reality, including human society: in Spencer's writings, "biological, human and social development are seen to constitute stages in one broad evolutionary continuum, subject to the same immutable laws and impelled by the same natural forces."[34] From the viewpoint of the more compartmentalized intellectual production of the twentieth- (or even late nineteenth-) century such aspirations appeared so grandiose as to be ridiculous. Spencer the systematist is, therefore, to be dismissed.

Jackson's endeavors have, in contrast, been treated with greater respect: they are, indeed, accorded the status of real science. Head recognized that his hero's Spencerian links were something of an embarrassment to those who wished to award this accolade to Jackson; but so long as these associations were seen as limited to a few, albeit key, concepts drawn from the more strictly biological part of Spencer's output the damage to Jackson's reputation could be limited. The fact that Spencer's biology was inseparable from a wider vision of reality is overlooked or deemed irrelevant.

If we abandon an exclusive reliance on such notions as "influence," "borrowing," and "use," and look instead for homologous discursive structures within the two sets of writings, a more comprehensive view of their affinity emerges. Both texts share a set of values that are constitutive of their factual content. The advantage of reading Jackson's texts in this comparative perspective is that what is implicit or occluded in his writing is often overt in that of Spencer. Authorship of these values cannot, how-

---

[32] For Jackson's own acknowledgment of this "debt" see his: "Evolution and Dissolution of the Nervous System," *Lancet* 1 (1884): 555–558, 649–652, 739–744, p. 555.

[33] For accounts of Spencer's thought see: J. D. Y. Peel, *Herbert Spencer: The Evolution of a Sociologist* (New York: Basic Books, 1971); David Wiltshire, *The Social and Political Thought of Herbert Spencer* (Oxford: Oxford University Press, 1978).

[34] Wiltshire, *Social and Political Thought*, p. 225.

ever, be ascribed to Spencer; he merely reinscribed some of the fundamental and unquestioned assumptions of his culture about the order of things.

In Spencer's account of the evolution of the "higher" mental powers, "the development of what we call Will, is but another aspect of the general process whose other aspects have been delineated in the last three chapters. Memory, Reason, and Feeling, simultaneously arise as the automatic actions become complex, infrequent, and hesitating; and Will, arising at the same time, is necessitated by the same conditions."[35] In keeping with his general uniformitarianism, Spencer did not therefore depict the origins of volition in terms of the appearance of some radically new entity; will emerged as a result of novel levels of complexity among pre-existing elements. He maintained that:

> When the automatic actions become so involved . . . as no longer to be performed with unhesitating precision—when, after the reception of one or more complex impressions, the appropriate motor changes become nascent, but are prevented from passing into immediate action by the antagonism of certain other nascent motor changes appropriate to some nearly allied impression; there is constituted a state of consciousness which, when it finally issues in action, displays what we term volition.[36]

"Will" was therefore something which emerged from below rather than an autocratic entity imposed upon the basal mental and nervous processes from above.

What distinguished a voluntary from an involuntary movement was merely that: "whereas the involuntary one occurs without previous consciousness of the movement to be made, the voluntary one occurs only after it has been represented in consciousness; and as the representation of it is nothing else than a weak form of the psychical state accompanying the movement, it is nothing else than a nascent excitation of the nerves concerned, preceding their actual excitation."[37]

This unemphatic, demystified account of the origins of the volitional belies, however, the significance Spencer subsequently places on this emergent property of nervous evolution. He held that the process whereby actions became less automatic as they became more complex was to be numbered among the "leading traits of developed intelligence, as distinguished from intelligence which is undeveloped."[38] The emergence of increasingly volitional action was thus depicted as a *goal* or endpoint of the

---

[35] Herbert Spencer, *The Principles of Psychology*, 2 vols. (London: Williams and Norgate, 1870), vol. 1, p. 495.
[36] Ibid., p. 496.
[37] Ibid., p. 497.
[38] Ibid., p. 580.

evolutionary process; thereby it acquired normative as well as merely descriptive properties.

It provided, in particular, a criterion for discriminating between "different grades of men":

> those having well-developed nervous systems will display a relatively-marked premeditation—an habitual representation of more various possibilities of cause, and conduct, and consequence—a greater tendency to suspense of judgments and an easier modification of judgments that have been formed. Those having nervous systems less developed, with fewer and simpler sets of connexions among their plexuses, will show less of hesitation—will be prone to premature conclusions that are difficult to change.[39]

"Well" and "less" developed nervous systems were therefore deemed equivalent to higher and lower kinds of man. The definitive characteristic of the "higher" human type was his propensity to deliberate and reflect before embarking upon any action; he was a prudent, rational, and responsible being—not unlike the model of a perfect Victorian gentleman.

The difference between "civilized" and "uncivilized" races was, for instance, essentially a matter of how closely they approximated to the volitional type. Spencer drew a contrast between "the comparatively-judicial intellect of the civilized man" and the tendency of the primitive mind to be "sudden in its inferences, incapable of balancing evidence, and adhering obstinately to first impressions." A similar, though less marked, difference was apparent "between the modes of thought of men and women; for women are the more quick to draw conclusions, and retain more pertinaciously the beliefs once formed." Even within the same race and gender it was possible to distinguish between the cultivated and uncultivated man or woman on the basis of varying capacities for deliberation and reasoned modification of conduct.[40]

The deliberative type was characterized by his ability to exercise control over the various and sometimes conflicting impulses arising in his consciousness. He was, therefore, *self*-disciplined. Spencer attached much significance to the evolution of this type of man as a precondition of societal amelioration; it required "no detail to show that a fundamental trait of social progress, is an increase of industrial energy, leading citizens to support themselves without being coerced in the harsh ways once general; that another fundamental trait is the gradual establishment of such a nature in citizens that, while pursuing their respective ends, they injure and impede one another in smaller degrees."[41] The history of civilization was

---

[39] Ibid., p. 581.
[40] Ibid., pp. 581–582.
[41] Herbert Spencer, *The Study of Sociology*, 17 ed. (London: Kegan Paul, 1894), p. 348.

in essence the chronicle of the molding of the loftiest forms of humanity into a form capable of such autoregulation and restraint. It was, in other words, the narrative of the emergence of economic and political liberalism as the highest forms of human social organization.

The importance of self-control as a cultural value and the emphasis upon the need for the higher (volitional) faculties to predominate over the lower (instinctual) has been discussed at length by Roger Smith in his study of the concept of inhibition, while Janet Oppenheim has considered the centrality of failure of the will in nineteenth-century British psychiatry with special reference to the emergent clinical entities of neurasthenia and depression.[42] Smith has, in particular, considered how this trope of "popular" psychology also structured aspects of the esoteric discourse of neurophysiology.[43] He has also shown that Jackson's debt to Spencer consisted of a biological idiom which permitted such blatantly evaluative distinctions to be introduced into the purported purely descriptive language of clinical medicine.[44]

I shall examine more especially Jackson's writings on aphasia with a view to uncovering the deep moral structures inherent in them. In so doing, I hope to draw attention to a number of features inherent in the dichotomous model of mind/brain on which Jackson relied that an exclusive emphasis on its obvious preoccupation with hierarchy and control may obscure. This is to insist that, as well as the overt and self-proclaimed metaphors to be found in Jackson's texts, there exists a more subtle and pervasive figural language. While the former may be dismissed as mere dispensable auxiliaries to the expression of ideas, the latter are inseparable from the conceptual core of his writing.[45]

I also hope to show that the role of cultural values in the emergence of pathologies, to which Oppenheim and others have drawn attention, is not confined to what may be classed as "soft" psychological disturbances. For most of the nineteenth century "nervous diseases" encompassed conditions which later came to be distinguished into those with a predomi-

---

[42] Janet Oppenheim, *"Shattered Nerves": Doctors, Patients, and Depression in Victorian England* (New York: Oxford University Press, 1991), especially pp. 43–44, 296–297.

[43] Roger Smith, *Inhibition: History and Meaning in the Sciences of Mind and Brain* (London: Free Association Books, 1992), especially chapter 4.

[44] Ibid., pp. 164–166.

[45] For a discussion of the suppression of the figurative contribution to rational discourse see: Christopher Norris, *Deconstruction: Theory and Practice* (London: Routledge, 1991), pp. 57–58. The imputation of a "merely" or improperly figural status to an opponent's language could, of course, serve polemical purposes—as, for instance, when Head complained that: "Neurology has become frozen stiffly in the grip of pseudo-metaphorical classifications which neither explain the conditions nor correspond to the clinical facts." "Hughlings Jackson," p. 3. Head's emphasis upon the rigorous descriptive purity of Jackson's neurological language needs to be viewed as a proposed alternative to such figurative laxity.

nantly mental component, which were the province of psychiatry, and those which were true neurological disorders. Although aphasia clearly possessed characteristics that might place it in either category, it was ultimately deemed to belong to neurology. Jackson's writing shows how cultural values were constitutive of even this hardwired pathology.

The Predicament of the Speechless Man

It is easy enough to find metaphors of government and vertical regulation in Jackson's writings.[46] The most striking of these occur in the Croonian Lectures on the "Evolution and Dissolution of the Nervous System" that he delivered in 1884. Here he developed an elaborate comparison between the workings of the highest nervous centers and the actions of an administrative agency—namely, the Naval Board. His concern was to show the supposed analogy between the direct and collateral effects of a pathologically discharging nervous center and the results of one member of the Board going insane and issuing "foolish orders" to his colleagues.[47]

Elsewhere in the lectures he gave further evidence of a concern to show the affinities between a highly evolved nervous system and a well-regulated polity. In the course of evolution there was a gradual adding on of new nervous organizations;

> But this "adding on" is at the time a "keeping down." The higher nervous arrangements evolved out of the lower keep down those lower, just as a government evolved out of a nation controls as well as directs that nation.

There was, however, a disturbing corollary to this conclusion:

> If this be the process of evolution, then the reverse process of dissolution is not only a "taking off" of the higher, but is at the very same time a "letting go" of the lower. If the governing body of this country were destroyed suddenly we should have two causes for lamentation: (1) The loss of services of eminent men; and (2) the anarchy of the now uncontrolled people.[48]

These men were "eminent" inasmuch as they approximated closely to the most fully evolved, deliberative human type.

This attention to the consequences of dissolution was a still more prominent feature of Jackson's writing than his account of the progressive evo-

---

[46] For a general discussion of the role of metaphor in neuroscience see: C. U. M. Smith, "The Use and Abuse of Metaphors in the History of Brain Science," *Journal of the History of the Neurosciences* 2 (1993): 283–301.

[47] Jackson, "Evolution," p. 649.

[48] Ibid., p. 651.

lution of nervous function. Although the highest (because most recently evolved) nervous centres exerted a legitimate sovereignty over the lower, older structures, their rule was fragile in the extreme. The machinery of the baser instincts remained intact and ready to resume its untrammeled activity at the first opportunity.

Aphasia and its kindred disorders provided the outstanding exemplification both of the fragility of the volitional man and of what remained after the higher centers were incapacitated by disease or injury.[49] In the extreme case of complete speechlessness, Jackson maintained, "There is a loss of intellectual (the more voluntary) language, with persistence of emotional (the more automatic) language."[50] The "speechless man" was therefore not silent but emitted a depraved form of language.

The coupling of the intellectual and voluntary as the antithesis of the automatic and emotional is of special significance. The corollary of the privileging of the volitional and deliberative was a deprecation of the emotional and spontaneous. Spencer maintained that the emotions were also subject to a progressive evolution, which rendered them more refined— quasi-intellectual—and less spontaneous. As a result, "along with advancing evolution of feelings there will go a diminution of fitfulness and uncertainty of conduct." Here, as in the case of the development of volition, there was a marked difference between the higher and lower races of humanity, while "a further but less marked illustration is furnished by the contrast between men and women."[51] Continued subjection to emotional impulse was thus a feminine trait. The female will was notoriously weaker than that of the male.

At an early stage in his writing on the disorders of speech Jackson adopted Spencer's view that "our muscles may be used in two kinds of language, one intellectual and the other emotional."[52] By means of the latter "we show what we feel, and by the other we tell what we think."[53] The relative value attached to these two forms of language was clear: only intellectual language qualified as the medium of genuine speech; emotional language was merely a form of involuntary ejaculation, of which swearing constituted the type. Jackson maintained that:

> Although oaths differ from mere alterations of tone, in that they consist of *articulate words*, they are generally used in talking, not to express ideas, but to make up by vigour in delivery what is wanting in precision of expression.

[49] On this point see: Smith, *Inhibition*, p. 49.

[50] Jackson, "Evolution," p. 556.

[51] Spencer, *Psychology*, vol. 1, p. 583.

[52] John Hughlings Jackson, "Clinical Remarks on Emotional and Intellectual Language in some Cases of Disease of the Nervous System [1866]," in "Reprint," 43–47, p. 46.

[53] Jackson, "Notes . . . Language," p. 48.

They may, indeed, be considered as phrases which emotion has filched from the intellect, to express itself in more definite terms than it could do by mere violence of tone or manner.[54]

Emotion was thus a thief who stole and misused the words that were the intellect's proper mode of expression.

The involuntary service of words was also to be disparaged because of its proximity to the corporeal. The interjections of which it consisted were "not speech, and take low rank in language, little above that of bodily starts, parts of common emotional language." Like other automatic bodily acts these utterances were highly organized and therefore immutable.[55] In contrast, the voluntary service of words was highly labile and therefore adapted to the changing needs of the intellect. In short, the emotional use of words was invariably a "more automatic, inferior utterance."[56]

Despite these sharp dichotomies, Jackson recognized a continuum between the various forms of utterance: the highest form of emotional language and the lowest form of the intellectual tended to merge. In the healthy subject the presence of the automatic service of words was, moreover, a precondition for the voluntary exercise of intellectual speech. On the physiological side, each type of language had its appropriate seat in the dominant and subordinate hemisphere of the brain repectively. The latter was, in particular, the site of a struggle between competing images, the "fittest" of which was then available to mentation.[57] Something akin to the state of nature therefore obtained in the subordinate hemisphere.

What rendered the condition of the aphasic so degrading was that he was left with *only* the inferior of the two services of words. In consequence, he was deprived of all the attributes that qualified him as an intellectual subject. Such a "man's mind" was, firstly, characterized by loss of his wilful capacities along with a concomitant heightening of the "minor or lower" side of his linguistic nature:[58] "the speechless man is seen to have lost the most voluntary or special part of language (speech), and not to have lost the more automatic language of emotional manifestation. He is in this way reduced to a more automatic condition of language." He became subject to the uncontrolled emission of these utterances at the same time

---

[54] Jackson, "Loss of Speech," p. 40.

[55] John Hughlings Jackson, "On Affections of Speech from Disease of the Brain [1880]," in "Reprint," 130–146, pp. 139–140.

[56] John Hughlings Jackson, "On Affections of Speech from Disease of the Brain [1880]," in "Reprint," 147–174, p. 163.

[57] Jackson, "Of Affections," p. 151.

[58] John Hughlings Jackson, "On Affections of Speech from Disease of the Brain [1879]," in "Reprint," 107–129, p. 118.

as he lost the power to "propositionize"—that is, to make *use* of language as his instrument. Because such utterances might be provoked by "wide bodily states," the speechless man ceased to be a sovereign subject and was at the mercy of his own corporeality.[59] A state of anarchy obtained within his cerebrum.

It is in this context that the full import of Jackson's image of the aphasic as "victim" emerges. Because he was not entirely wordless but merely speechless, he could be made to suffer the propositional acts of another. He had reverted to an infantile condition: the aphasic's state was equivalent to "that of the little child which has been taught to understand speech, and has not yet spoken."[60] The speechless man was, in effect, rendered passive, impotent, feminine.[61]

Others were to judge his utterances accordingly; they would not give whatever words he might still be able to articulate "the credit of being propositions."[62] Even when they possessed a proper propositional form, they were "intellectually dead."[63] Such ejaculations were merely "interjections, not speech, and take a low rank in language, little above that of bodily starts, parts of common emotional language. At the best they are propositions, entirely subordinated to the service of an emotion." A further characteristic of these emissions was their "highly organized"—that is, predetermined—nature.[64] They lacked the spontaneity that distinguished the intellectual use of language, and which was among the defining attributes of the autonomous subject. The speechless man "must utter" whatever jargon was left to him irrespective of the context in which he found himself.[65]

The anatomical correlate of this psychic degradation consisted in the abeyance of the operations of the active side of the brain accompanied by the survival of (in evolutionary terms) lower nervous processes located in the right hemisphere. The right hemisphere was thus identified, in conformity to a well-established system of binary oppositions, with the more "natural," feminine side of personality.[66]

---

[59] John Hughlings Jackson, "On the Nature of the Duality of the Brain [1874]," in "Reprint," 87–95, p. 89. For Jackson's notion of propositionizing see: Jackson, "On Affections," pp. 113–114.

[60] Ibid., p. 127.

[61] This image of the aphasic as child was widely disseminated: see chapter 7.

[62] Jackson, "On Affections," p. 136.

[63] Ibid., p. 147.

[64] Ibid., pp. 139–140.

[65] Ibid., p. 158.

[66] On the identification of the feminine with the natural see Ludmilla Jordanova, *Sexual Visions: Images of Gender in Science and Medicine between the Eighteenth and Twentieth Centuries* (New York: Harvester Wheatsheaf, 1989), pp. 41–42. In her study of the double brain concept, Harrington, recognizes that the two hemispheres were ascribed "gender identities"

A comparison between Jackson's speechless man and Spencer's notion of the difference between male and female psychic attributes is instructive. Just as women's bodies were more childlike than those of men so their minds displayed distinguishing characteristics resulting "from a somewhat-earlier arrest of individual evolution in women than in men." In consequence of this arrested development women fell short in the highest forms of human intellectual and emotional attainment.[67]

Women were, for instance, more apt "to dwell on the concrete and proximate rather than on the abstract and remote." But the feminine was also marked by a greater tendency to *dependence* and subordination when compared with the autonomy characteristic of the masculine:

> Faith in whatever presents itself with imposing accompaniments, is . . . especially strong in women. Doubt, or criticism, or calling-in-question of things that are established, is rare among them. Hence in public affairs their influence goes towards the maintenance of controlling agencies, and does not resist the extension of such agencies. Reverencing power more than men do, women, by implication, respect freedom less—freedom, that is, not of the nominal kind, but of that real kind which consists in the ability of each to carry on his own life without hindrance from others, so long as he does not hinder them.[68]

Women were therefore, in Jackson's sense, more "organized"; they were, in consequence, natural victims.

For an advocate of liberal individualism like Spencer the natural propensities of women carried a negative moral charge. Their social influence militated against the autonomous and spontaneous exercise of human faculties that was the effective telos of the evolutionary process. The most distinctively feminine attributes were also the most morally and politically retrograde: not only were women susceptible to manipulation, they were inherently conservative.

John Hughlings Jackson was not a social philosopher; he did not articulate any political theory in his writings. This is not, however, to say that his works are value-free and politically neutral. A particular evaluative concept of human nature pervaded his textual work as it had that of Spencer. This was the source of those dead, because unrecognized, metaphors that underlay his account of the workings of the mind/brain. There was, moreover, an isomorphism between the allocation of worth within this system

---

with the right being perceived as embodying female traits; she identifies this as an example of "how the language and imagery of science and medicine may unconsciously be used by society to express and sanction certain of its cultural 'truths.' " *Medicine*, pp. 88–89, 100. She fails, however, to apply these insights in her analysis of Jackson's writing.

[67] Spencer, *Sociology*, pp. 373–374.
[68] Ibid., p. 380.

and the distribution of power within his society. The metaphorical system he deployed made it possible "to build up a pyramidal order with castes and grades, to create a new world of laws privileges, suborders, delimitations."[69]

Jackson operated with a notion of the normal, optimal "man;" nervous disease was represented as a deviation from or deformation of this type. In particular, aphasia was depicted as an encroachment upon man's volitional, self-determining aspect: as an insult to the intellectual subject. It therefore impinged upon the defining characteristics of the protagonist of liberal, possessive individualism. Jackson's clinical histories are, overtly, gender blind; in many of his cases the "speechless man" is, in fact, a woman. Spencer's writings display more clearly that the human norm was deemed to be masculine in character; the feminine was necessarily pathological because it constituted a failure to attain to this ideal. The pathos of the predicament of the speechless man lay precisely in the fact that his affliction brought him perilously close to woman's natural estate.

Conclusion

Henry Head celebrated Jackson's writing on aphasia for its modest and unassuming aspect. Paradoxically such humility in the face of nature had led to profound insights of lasting value. In contrast to contemporaries who felt it necessary to discipline cases by means of diagrammatic schemata, Jackson was supposed to have allowed clinical experience to speak— or not—for itself. Head especially commended Jackson's willingness to explore the psychological aspects of these complaints; from the vantage point of his bridge, he surveyed the stream of consciousness in order to explicate the subjective aspect of the aphasic condition.

But as soon as he came to verbalize his observations, Jackson necessarily entered the realm of discourse; in order to say what he had seen and heard, he was obliged to draw upon the repertoires of representation available in his culture. He relied, in particular, upon the resources of the linguistic regime of introspective analysis: his protagonist became the transcendental ego of the metaphysician. The lineaments of this subject were accordingly shaped by the polarities and discriminations inherent in this form of discourse. Its essence comprised its capacity for deliberative, willed action; conversely, the "emotional" was bracketed with the automatic as forming the inferior stratum of human personality.

Evolutionary biology provided a temporal ordering for these dualisms. The intellectual and volitional were "higher" because they were the latest

---

[69] Nietzsche, "Of Truth and Falsity," p. 181.

products of the developmental process evident in nature. The anatomical substrates of the mental powers in the human nervous system were regulated accordingly: normally, the emotional and instinctual centers were inhibited in their actions by the reflective processes of the cerebral cortex. Even at this level, however, dualism and subordination persisted: the dominant hemisphere embodied the volitional type of action more fully than its more affective and automatic partner.

Any discursive practice so heavily implicated in questions of difference and precedence necessarily incorporated the asymmetries ascribed to gender. The metaphysical subject was masculine in its disembodiment and—at least putatively—in its purely intellectual identity. Language was the instrument of its expression and projection into the external world. One advantage of reading Jackson's and Spencer's writings as different chapters of a *single* text is that the latter make explicit the gendered nature of the type of human normality that was immanent in the former.

Jackson's account of aphasia is, therefore, very much the tragedy of the speechless *man*. The condition is rendered as an encroachment on precisely those powers that define the normal subject. The impairment of those faculties by brain disease was tantamount to emasculation. His vision of the nervous system incorporated, not only a vertical hierarchy, but also a lateral duality that corresponded to this binary concept of human nature.

It is an apparent paradox that Jackson's writing also embodies—as has been widely recognized—a marked preoccupation with continuity; it is distinguished by its refusal to respect some of the most deeply trenched bifurcations of Western culture. At the same time that he insisted upon a strict separation between psychological and physiological language, he assimilated what was conventionally designated as purely intellectual to the category of bodily acts. Jackson supposed "the nervous system to be a sensori-motor mechanism, from bottom to top; that every part of the nervous system represents impressions or movements, or both." The highest centers, which formed the physical basis of consciousness were no exception to this law as was shown by their genealogy: "they are evolved out of the middle, as the middle are out of the lowest, and the lowest are out of the periphery."[70]

Although they were the "organ of mind," these centers "are 'for body' too; strictly they are for nothing else—for nothing else than for co-ordinating or representing the different parts of the body."[71] It followed that the most elevated operations of the brain were not different in essence from the more mundane sensori-motor functions. For example, "centres

[70] Jackson, "Remarks on Evolution," pp. 29–30.
[71] Ibid., p. 36.

for movements of the tongue, palate, lips, &c., as concerned in eating, swallowing, &c., are in the highest centres evolved into the physical bases of words, symbols serving us during abstract reasoning."[72]

Such stress upon the mundane motor nature of speech acts has an obvious affinity to the attempts to demystify language by demonstrating the organic conditions of its exercise discussed in chapter 2. Jackson occasionally identified with the tenets of scientific naturalism—the nearest English analogue of French positivism. "The evolutionist," he declared, "does not . . . invoke supernatural agency." Monism could, moreover, be sanctioned on purely pragmatic grounds: "Our concern as medical men is with the body. If there be such a thing as disease of the mind, we can do nothing for it."[73]

While certain categorical boundaries were subverted others, however, remained intact. So deeply embedded were they in the language of analysis available to Jackson that their existence and their evaluative and discriminating function was invisible. The same texts that, in one register, challenged the traditional distinction between the mental and the physical remained conservative as to the constitution of mind and its relation to the bodily.

But an insistence upon the principle of continuity did challenge the permanence and stability of the polarities and hierarchies between reason and emotion, volitional and automatic, masculine and feminine. For Jackson—as for Spencer—the highest form of emotional action and the lowest form of the voluntary were virtually indistinguishable. Moreover, his pathology provided an extended disquisition upon how easily these categorical distinctions could collapse through neurological disorder to produce a linguistic eunuch.[74]

Henry Head's representation of Jackson's place in the history of aphasia studies has served here as a starting point for an examination of the silences and fractures in the latter's texts. In particular, Head's analysis is valuable for specifying what is most distinctive in Jackson's writing: namely, that, in contrast with most of his contemporaries, he sought to understand the condition of speechlessness *from within*. This opened up a space in which to speculate upon the inner world of the aphasic: to imagine, for instance, the extent to which a patient retained the power to "propositionize," to make utterances that represented the will of a rational being. The answer given to this question was not merely of theoretic inter-

---

[72] Ibid., p. 48.

[73] Ibid., pp. 38–39.

[74] It is possible, though for the purposes of my argument not obligatory, to place this representation of the fragility of the masculine subject in the context of later nineteenth-century preoccupation with the nature of "manliness" and the threat of encroaching effeminacy. See: Jordanova, *Sexual Visions*, p. 22.

est; it could determine whether an individual remained master of his or her own affairs.[75]

Head's depiction of Jackson needs, however, also to be viewed as a rhetorical gesture calculated to produce certain effects. It formed part of an extensive assault upon the legacy of classical aphasiology in which the history of the subject served as a polemical weapon. In this context, it was expedient to seek founding, precursory figures for a self-consciously new neurology: to show "how closely Jackson had arrived at the sort of position we hold to-day."[76] Although *of* the past, Jackson was active *in* the present. The incomprehension and neglect of his ideas by Jackson's contemporaries helped to emphasize the interval separating the putatively modern from the allegedly archaic.

[75] See the avowedly Jacksonian discussion of testamentary capacity in: R. Percy Smith, "Aphasia in Relation to Mental Disease," *Proceedings of the Royal Society of Medicine* 11 (1917–18): 1–20.

[76] Henry Head to Charles Sherrington, 8 October 1925, Sherrington MSS, 00570, Department of Physiology, Oxford.

FIVE

HEAD WOUNDS

To refrain from mutual injury, mutual violence, mutual
exploitation, to equate one's own will with that of another:
this may in a certain rough sense become good manners
between individuals if the conditions for it are present
(namely if their strength and value standards are in fact
similar and they both belong to *one* body).
(Friedrich Nietzsche, Beyond Good and Evil, *§ 259)*

T HE FIRST and third chapters of this book have described the
emergence in the nineteenth century of a linguistic technology
serviceable to the requirements of a science of aphasia. The chief
characteristics of this genre of case history was the construction of the
patient as object of the medical gaze; an object whose own perspective and
narrative capacities were strictly circumscribed, if not entirely suppressed,
in the name of clinical relevance. The patient was, in short, denied any
authorial role in the creation of his or her history. There was, indeed, some
question as to whether the clinical narrative *was* "his" story, as opposed
to a narrative whose subject was man, his brain, and its diseases. At its
limits, the discourse of aphasia sought to reduce this narrative to a matter
of purely spatial relations: a set of coordinates imprinted upon the surface
of "the brain" amenable to schematic exposition.

We have already seen how at the turn of the twentieth century certain
aspects of aphasiology became controversial. The adequacy and worth of
its most distinctive mode of representation, the diagram, attracted especial
criticism. In this chapter I wish to examine more closely the writings of
one of the most trenchant of these critics, the British neurologist Henry
Head. I will, in particular, seek to scrutinize the *textual* consequences of
his avowed departure from the norms of previous work on aphasia.

I shall also consider the way in which Head sought to overcome the
perceived obstacles in the way of an adequate understanding of aphasia by
recruiting allies who possessed special forms of expertise. Foremost among
the assistants who were allowed a voice in Head's narrative were the aphasics themselves. Following Bruno Latour, I have, however, also allowed
for the possibility of Head's recruitment of nonhuman allies.[1]

---

[1] The allusion is to the argument of Bruno Latour, *The Pasteurization of France* (Cambridge, Mass.: Harvard University Press, 1988). This borrowing is limited, however, to the

Henry Head was born in north London in 1861 into a Quaker family. He was distantly related to the surgeon, Joseph Lister, and recalled in his autobiography that: "I was brought up in an atmosphere of modern science and in an attitude of worship for the great man who was connected with my own people."[2] He was educated at Charterhouse and then spent some time at the University of Halle before proceeding to Trinity College, Cambridge where he read for the natural sciences Tripos. He attended Michael Foster's physiology lectures as well as attending practical classes conducted by J. N. Langley and Sheridan Lea; it was at this time that he also became acquainted with W. H. Gaskell, who was "just beginning his fundamental researches on the Heart, and from the first his geniality and enthusiasm captured our imagination." As a precocious demonstrator in the physiology department, Head was "brought into intimate contact with the active research carried on by both Gaskell and Langley."[3]

Foster apparently dissuaded Head temporarily from his original intention of following a career in medicine and encouraged him to pursue his interest in laboratory science.[4] To this end, Head for two years studied physiology in Prague with Ewald Hering. On his return to Cambridge, however, he reverted to his original plan of qualifying in and practicing medicine. But a scientific bent derived from his early training in laboratory science left its mark upon his approach to clinical questions.

Head's clinical training took place at University College Hospital in London. Head subsequently held various junior hospital posts before his appointment to the staff of the London Hospital to which he remained attached until the end of his career. During his early London years Head became acquainted with the neurologist John Hughlings Jackson whose (at that time) unconventional ideas on aphasia (see chapter 4) were later to make a great impression on his own work in the subject.

Head had shown an early leaning towards the study of the nervous system and its ailments: his MD dissertation had been "On Disturbances of Sensation, with Special Reference to the Pain of Visceral Disease." Normal and pathological sensation was to figure largely in Head's later researches. He was, most notably, his own experimental subject in a series of inquiries on the consequences of the sectioning and regeneration of cutaneous nerves undertaken at Saint John's College, Cambridge in collaboration

---

suggestion that additional insights may be gleaned by seeking nonhuman agents in the texts under consideration.

[2] "Autobiography of Henry Head," Contemporary Medical Archive Centre (CMAC), Wellcome Institute for the History of Medicine, PP HEA, Box 1, p. 4.

[3] Ibid., pp. 31, 34. For an account of these researches and of the Cambridge context more generally see Gerald L. Geison, *Michael Foster and the Cambridge School of Physiology: The Scientific Enterprise in Late Victorian Society* (Princeton: Princeton University Press, 1978).

[4] Ibid., p. 34.

with W. H. R. Rivers.[5] Later Head also published the results of his investigations on disorders of sensation arising from damage to the cerebral cortex and thalamus. There was a strong element of continuity in approach and method between these studies and Head's later work on aphasia.

Aphasia: Before and After

Head's special interest in aphasic disorders seems to have been sparked by a reading of John Hughlings Jackson's numerous writings on the subject.[6] In an attempt to make these texts more accessible, Head in 1915 reprinted them in the neurological journal *Brain* (see chapter 4). In 1920 Head delivered the John Hughlings Jackson Lecture, choosing "Aphasia: An Historical Review" as his subject. In the same year he took the opportunity of another public lecture to present for the first time the results of his own investigations on aphasia. In 1926 a much expanded version of these lectures appeared as a two volume work entitled *Aphasia and Kindred Disorders of Speech*.

Head's history of aphasia studies provided a highly partisan account of how, in the author's view, the great bulk of the work on aphasia that had appeared since the 1860s had been misguided and had yielded results that actually militated against any real understanding of the clinical manifestations and pathological correlates of these disorders. "It is generally conceded," he wrote in 1925, "that the views on aphasia and analogous disturbances of speech found in the text-books of to-day are of little help in understanding an actual case of disease."[7]

Previous aphasiologists were at fault partly in the concepts of brain function with which they operated. They took the view that high-order functions like language could be analysed into component sensory and motor acts each of which occurred at a determinate site on the cerebral cortex. Aphasia was to be understood as the consequence of the disruption of one or more of these sensori-motor operations as a result of injury to

---

[5] These researches were reprinted as: W. H. R. Rivers and Henry Head, "A Human Experiment in Nerve Division," in Henry Head, *Studies in Neurology*, 2 vols. (London: Hodder and Stoughton), vol. 1, pp. 225–323.

[6] Head had, however, taken an interest in aphasia from a much earlier date. He wrote in 1901 of a patient who "in consequence of a blow on the head has entirely lost the visual element in speech but is otherwise quite normal." Letter to Ruth Mayhew, 13[?] January 1901, CMAC, PP HEA D4/8. The suggestion that this patient had lost only a discrete portion of his linguistic capacity while retaining the remainder is, however, scarcely compatible with Head's later holism.

[7] Henry Head, "Hughlings Jackson on Aphasia and Kindred Affections of Speech," *Brain* 38 (1915): 1–190, on p. 1.

one of these so-called "language centers" or to the nervous commissures that existed between them.

In the classical phase of aphasia studies elaborate diagrams were generated, which purported to represent these anatomical and functional relations (see chapter 3). One could supposedly predict from one of these diagrams what clinical manifestations would result from damage to any given part of this circulation. Conversely it was possible to infer from a patient's symptoms which part of the brain was injured. Head objected to the excessive rationalism of this project: its tendency to privilege the mind's desire for order over the intractability of the facts to tidy classification. His rhetoric emphasized the clinician's responsibility to be faithful in his writing to the particularity of the case rather than an overriding obligation to discover the typical essence underlying a singular event.

Head is generally included in what has been called the holist movement in early twentieth-century neurology. He maintained that the notion of circumscribed "centers" on the cortex in which discrete functions were located was misguided. He was not opposed to the concept of cerebral localization as such, but, along with his friend the physiologist Charles Sherrington, he held that a much looser, more dynamic, understanding was required of how particular sensations and movements were represented at the highest levels of the nervous system.

Moreover, Head challenged the view that language could be understood as a mixture of sensory and motor operations. He resisted the reductionism inherent in earlier aphasia studies. He argued instead that high-level actions of this kind could only be understood in terms of the function itself. The mark of the true scientist was his readiness to let the phenomena speak for themselves in their own dialect rather than attempting to translate these events into some other tongue. Any attempt to classify the language disorders presenting in the clinic into such categories as "sensory," "motor," "affective," and "emissive" aphasias was, on this notion of scientific propriety, therefore utterly misguided.

Head reserved special scorn for the "diagram makers" such as H. Charlton Bastian. Their confident localizations of where in the brain the sensory and motor language centers were situated were vitiated by conceptual confusions; they did not even properly appreciate *what* it was they were trying to localize. All attempts at a pathological anatomy of aphasia had to wait upon an adequate classification of the syndromes grouped under this rubric themselves.

As well as these theoretical weaknesses Head also found fault with the investigative methods previous aphasiologists had employed; in truth, however, the two vices were inextricably linked. Clinical histories tended to be superficial, perfunctory, and tendentious: Head compared them to a procrustean bed upon which each case was either stretched or lopped to make it fit some preexisting schema. Classical aphasiology therefore mutilated nature to make her fit its preconceptions rather than providing a faithful representation of nature. There was, moreover, a failure to examine the diachronic element of these disorders: to see how a patient's linguistic capacities might alter over the entire course of his or her affliction. A mania for mapping and obsession with spatial relations had led to a neglect of narrative.

The dire state of aphasia studies before Head was therefore primarily the fault of past neurologists operating with inadequate techniques and with faulty and inappropriate concepts. These vices were epitomized in the flawed literary technology the science employed; Head's polemic was in large part a trenchant literary criticism. Besides Jackson, Head had little good to say for any of his predecessors in the field; Arnold Pick and Sigmund Freud were virtually the only ones whose writings on aphasia possessed any merit. Head's historiography therefore amounted to an extended and destructive critique of the received text of aphasiology. Apart from a few honorable and carefully bracketed exceptions, it was necessary to expunge what had been inscribed and to make a new beginning. Head thus sketched a role for himself to fill as an innovator and iconoclast who would set the world of aphasia studies on a sounder foundation.

But the fault also lay with the patients who had provided the "case material" for earlier authors on aphasia. The typical aphasic encountered in ordinary clinical experience possessed, Head insisted, serious shortcomings as an experimental subject. "In civilian practice," he declared, "many of those who suffer from aphasia are old, broken down in health and their general intellectual capacity is diminished." As well as these general characteristics, the particular nature of their lesions also diminished the value of these patients for scientific purposes: "Most of them are affected with arterial degeneration and in many the blood tension is greatly increased. Such patients are easily fatigued and are obviously unsuitable for sustained examination."[8] Progress in aphasia studies was therefore dependent not only upon a new kind of neurologist, but also upon the appearance of a different, more serviceable patient.

Finding the Ideal Patient

How can I serve who am too old to fight?
I cannot stand and wait
With folded hands and lay me down at night
In restless expectation that the day

---

[8] Henry Head, *Aphasia and Kindred Disorders of Speech*, 2 vols. (Cambridge: Cambridge University Press, 1926), vol. 1, p. 146.

Will bring some stroke of Fate
I cannot help to stay.
Once, like the spider in his patterned web,
Based on immutable law,
Boldly I spun the strands of arduous thought,
Now seeming nought,
Rent in the sudden hurricane of war.
Within my corner I will take my place,
And grant me grace
Some delicate thing to perfect and complete
With passionate contentment, as of old
Before my heart grew cold.
This in the Temple I will dedicate,
A widow's mite,
Among more spacious gifts, obscured from sight
By the majestic panoply of state.
But when triumphal candles have burnt low
And valorous trophies crumbled with dust
Perchance my gift may glow
Still radiating sacrificial joy
Amid the ravages of moth and dust.

(*Henry Head January 1915*)[9]

Head's own work on aphasia was predicated upon the availability of a very different class of patient. Nineteen fourteen was to prove a turning point in the history of aphasia studies. During the First World War Head abandoned his private practice in order to tend wounded soldiers admitted to the London Hospital; he also served at various convalescent hospitals dedicated to the care of wounded officers, notably the Empire Hospital at Vincent Square, Westminster. As the poem quoted above indicates, he evinced frustration at his inability to contribute directly to the war effort; by caring for the wounded he was able to assuage that guilt. He expressed the hope, moreover, that this work might produce a gift of abiding luminosity. Head's ardor could serve science as well as his nation.

Among the patients he encountered during and soon after the war were a number of aphasics whose aspect was quite different to those commonly encountered: Head wrote in 1926 that:

the war brought under our care young men who were struck down in the full pride of health. Many of them were extremely intelligent, willing and anxious to be examined thoroughly. As their wounds healed, they were encouraged and cheered by the obvious improvement in their condition. They were eu-

[9] The poem was sent to Charles Sherrington and is now among the Sherrington papers in the Department of Physiology at Oxford.

phoric rather than depressed, and in every way contrasted with the state of the aphasic met with in civilian practice.[10]

Head's admiration for these men is evident from this passage; in private, he expressed affection describing them as "these dear young men."[11] These wounded soldiers—and, above all, the wounded *officers* Head treated—were the first of the allies Head recruited to his cause.

The injuries with which these soldiers were afflicted were, in a sense, also Head's allies: these lesions were, he alleged, peculiarly suited to the needs of someone seeking a basic classification of the types of aphasic disorder. Gunshot wounds of the head tended to produce as their immediate aftermath massive and diffuse symptoms. Head invoked Constantin von Monakow's (1853–1930) concept of diaschisis[12] in order to distinguish between these transient sequelae and the more permanent impairment of function following a particular injury to the brain. Head argued that in a typical case of gunshot wound

> the symptoms tend to clear up to a considerable extent, provided there are no secondary complications, even though the effect produced by the initial impact of the bullet may have been extremely severe. Some aspects of the disordered functions of speech recover more rapidly than others and the clinical manifestations assume more or less characteristic forms. . . . By this means we are enabled to trace the various steps by which the defective functions are restored, whereas in civilian practice any change in the clinical manifestations is usually in an opposite direction.[13]

In other words, while the cerebral lesions that typically gave rise to aphasic symptoms in civilian practice were prone to grow more complicated over time, aphasias caused by gunshot wounds tended in the course of their natural history to become *simpler* and therefore more instructive.

But it is important to stress that for Head the patients whom he studied were much more than bodies bearing a certain kind of injury. He followed Hughlings Jackson's lead and insisted on the necessity of understanding aphasic disorders as psychological as well as anatomical or merely behavioral phenomena. Indeed, he seemed to see such an emphasis upon the patient's subjective experience as one of the defining features of the new neurology that was emerging in the aftermath of the First World War. Head placed these developments in the context of a widespread revision

---

[10] Head, *Aphasia*, vol. 1, p. 146.

[11] Letter to Ruth Head, 25 March 1917, CMAC PP HEAD D4/19.

[12] Von Monakow used "diaschisis" to refer to the diffuse but transitory symptoms that followed some shock to the brain: "Lokalisation der Hirnfunktionen," *Journal für Psychologie und Neurologie* 17 (1911): 185–200.

[13] Ibid.

of values occurring in the aftermath of this disaster. "The cataclysmic events of the last four years," he wrote in 1918, "have shaken men's belief in the old order, and medicine has not escaped the universal demand for a restatement of current values. The young are looking to us to enunciate the principles on which our teaching is founded."[14] Among these principles was a new attention to phenomena that a previous generation of neurologists would have considered "frivolous"; and these included "the importance attached to the patient's account of his own sensations, or the diagnostic value now attributed to certain dreams."[15]

Moreover, Head was not concerned with the patient solely as a perceptive being. He argued for the need to endow the patient with a "personality"—to see him (very rarely her) as a being with established capacities and possessing a unique life history. Aphasia studies were to be regarded as part of "the psychology of the concrete individual."[16] The literary products of aphasiology must be equal to this conception of the scope of the subject; the flimsy sketches of the patient typical of an earlier genre of case history was no longer adequate. Especially when dealing with Head's preferred type of patient such writing was indeed *unworthy* of the subject.

Personality was, in large part, a matter of "intelligence." Head repeatedly insisted that one of the advantages of his officer-patients was that they possessed sufficient intelligence and capacity to understand the nature of the tests being performed upon them, and indeed to participate in the process of inquiry in an active and creative way. He remarked of one case, for instance, that "the clinical observations were of unusual completeness and interest owing to the great intelligence of the patient," as well as to the fact that Head had the opportuinty of examining this individual over a period of more than four years.[17]

The mood of these examinations was, Head maintained, entirely different from that of cases involving "old and broken-down" civilian patients: "As their wounds healed they were encouraged and cheered by the obvi-

---

[14] Such drawing of sharp dichotomies between the world "before" and "after" the war was a typical trope of the period. See: Paul Fussell, *The Great War and Modern Memory* (London: Oxford University Press, 1975), chapter 3.

[15] Henry Head, "Some Principles of Neurology," *Lancet* 2 (1918): 657–660, on p. 657. Two of Head's collaborators, W. H. R. Rivers and G. Elliot Smith, were involved during the war in attempts to use the interpretation of dreams as an aid in the treatment of psychoneuroses. Smith wrote in 1922: "When Dr Rivers joined the staff of the Military Hospital at Maghull . . . in July 1915 he was introduced to a society in which the interpretation of dreams and the discussion of mental conflicts formed the staple subjects of conversation." G. Elliot Smith, "Preface," to W. H. R. Rivers, *Conflict and Dream* (London: Kegan Paul, 1923), pp. viii–ix. Smith was also on the staff at Maghull at this time; see: Richard Slobodin, *W. H. R. Rivers* (New York: Columbia University Press, 1978), pp. 55–57.

[16] "Discussion on Aphasia," *Brain* 43 (1920): 412–450, on p. 445.

[17] Head, *Aphasia*, vol. 1, p. 456.

ous improvement in their condition. They were euphoric rather than depressed, and in every way contrasted profoundly with the state of the aphasic met with in civilian practice."[18] A series of polarities between the "old" and the "new" aphasic were thus established. The former was, indeed, old, the latter young; one was intelligent the other *obtuse*. The aphasic met with in civilian practice was in a state of degeneration; the officer-patient's condition was progressive. While the mood of the old aphasic was despondent, encounters with the new variety occurred in an atmosphere of "euphoria."

Head's ideal patients were as much his willing collaborators as his experimental subjects. It is in this context that his rejection of Pierre Marie's claim that aphasia was always accompanied by some diminution of the "general intellect" should be viewed; only a patient who, despite his linguistic disabilities, retained his general "intelligence" could fill the demanding role that Head envisaged.

Personality was not, however, solely a matter of intelligence. It was also structured by the patient's occupational and social status as well as by the form of medical practice in which he or she was encountered. In his earlier investigations on sensation Head had devoted some attention to the question of the relative experimental value of different types of patient. "The hospital patient," he maintained, "is frequently an admirable subject for sensory experiments; at his best he answers 'Yes' and 'No' with certainty, and is commendably steady under the fatigue of control experiments." These were not unlike the qualities demanded of a good enlisted man. Such patients could, however, "tell little or nothing of the nature of their sensations, and the time they are able, or willing, to give is insufficient for elaborate psycho-physical testing." In short, a patient who submitted to tests solely for "the cure of his disease" was of limited scientific value. Evidence demanding introspection was, in particular, not to be trusted from patients of any class; a "trained observer" was required.[19] It was for this reason that Head made himself the subject as well as observer of his experiments on cutaneous sensibility.

When it came to his investigations of aphasia Head adopted a somewhat different attitude. While few or none of the patients presenting with these conditions might qualify as trained observers, some of them were considered markedly more informative subjects and more reliable witnesses of their condition—and, in particular, of its introspective aspect—than others.

[18] Henry Head, "Aphasia and Kindred Disorders of Speech," *Brain* 43 (1920): 87–165, on pp. 90–91.
[19] Head, *Studies*, vol. 1, pp. 225–226.

One of the difficulties facing all attempts to estimate the extent and nature of language loss in any given case was, Head maintained, that the investigator was usually ignorant of the patient's linguistic capacities *before* his illness or injury. The officer-patients Head encountered during and after the war were constructed to overcome this obstacle to knowledge. Since

> it is impossible to discover how the patient would have responded before he became aphasic, I have depended mainly on the reactions of young men wounded in the war; for, especially in the case of officers, it was possible to estimate with considerable accuracy the extent of their education, and the ability with which they had carried out the more exacting of their military duties. At the same time the profession or occupation exercised before the war frequently showed that they must have possessed faculties which were found to be grossly affected.[20]

In other words, Head was able to gauge with confidence the linguistic deficit in these officer-patients because he knew how they *should* be able to speak, read, and write. And this familiarity with their normal symbolic performances rested upon the fact that these were the kind of men with whose conversation Head was familiar; they were the sort of men with whom he had mixed all his adult life; they were, in short, *gentlemen*. This ascription of status had important consequences for the form and content of Head's case histories.

Head was prepared to receive such patients as competent and reliable collaborators because they were deemed to possess something akin to what Simon Schaffer, writing of an earlier period, has called "the *Cartesianism of the genteel*: in polite society, members could be treated as capable of separating their disorderly bodies from the cool deliverances of their intellectual judgment."[21] But in this case it might be more apposite to speak of the *schizophrenia of the genteel*: a gentleman's supposed "self-possession"—his capacity to remain a trustworthy witness of the disorderly conduct of some damaged portion of his psyche. Non-commissioned patients, on the other hand, were denied this unquestioned capacity to separate what was normal from what was pathological in their minds. They were merely uniformed members of what Head had elsewhere called the "ordinary hospital class."[22]

In the course of a previous war Head had used the occasion of a visit to the Army Hospital at Netley to provide a detailed exposition of the various

---

[20] Head, *Aphasia*, vol. 1, p. 148.

[21] Simon Schaffer, "Self Evidence," *Critical Inquiry* 18 (1992): 327–362, pp. 338–339.

[22] Henry Head and James Sherren, "The Consequences of Injury to the Peripheral Nerves in Man," *Brain* 28 (1905): 117–338, on p. 286.

social "types" to be found in the armed forces. The Royal Army Medical Corps officers he encountered there impressed him: "Their friendliness was apparent and their manners had that pleasant ease which always charms me in the best kind of soldier." In contrast, the other ranks whom Head encountered in the hospital were depicted in a less favorable light. One (Irish) patient was "little more than a fine beast but a splendid soldier." Another, the son of "a workman in Margate," talked "with that curious precise drawl that this type assumes with no mistakes in grammar or pronunciation."[23] For the purposes of his work on sensation, such social, cultural, and linguistic distinctions were of merely incidental interest; when Head came to study aphasia, however, they attained a novel cognitive significance.

Head subjected his model patients to a battery of tests. He stressed both the need to examine the full range of an individual's capacity for symbolic expression and apprehension and the necessity of repeating these tests over an extended period in order to obtain a true case *history*. He followed the progress of some of his patients over a period of several years. A set of experiments of such extent and of such duration obviously depended not upon the mere acquiescence, but on the active commitment of the patient to the investigative enterprise.

This was notably the case with one of Head's civilian patients—"Dr. P"—whom one test "interested . . . greatly owing to his scientific training and he was anxious to discover on what this difference depended."[24] But his officer-patients also showed to a marked degree a readiness to participate actively in their examination; they were, Head noted, "anxious to be examined thoroughly."[25] They might even seek to supplement Head's own experiments with spontaneous contributions to the project. Thus, "during a set of observations, No. 14 suddenly exclaimed, 'Funny thing, this worse, that sort of thing,' and seizing his note-book wrote 'as, at.' I asked, 'You mean conjunctions and prepositions?' and he replied, 'Yes, that sort of thing.' "[26] Unlike Dr. P., these patients might not be scientists by training; their general education and innate intelligence however made them competent to participate in the investigative enterprise that centered on their own minds and bodies.

---

[23] Letter of 1 March [1902] to Ruth Mayhew, CMAC, PP HEA D4/11. Head was at Netley to examine patients with peripheral nerve injuries as part of his investigations into sensation.

[24] Head, *Aphasia*, vol. 1, p. 266.

[25] Henry Head, "Aphasia: An Historical Review," *Brain* #43 (1920): 390–450, on p. 403.

[26] Head, *Aphasia*, vol. 1, p. 230.

Technologies of Inquiry

The intimacy of the relationship between subject and examiner was heightened by the fact that the investigative procedure was to be tailored to each patient's individuality: "The order in which these observations are carried out and the character of the task selected must be strictly adapted to the intelligence and education of the patient and to the nature of his disability."[27] Results were also to be evaluated with reference to "personality." Thus in one instance Head noted that "No. 15 alone, a man of comparatively defective education, failed to carry out the hand, eye and ear tests to orders given in print."[28] On another occasion, when a patient's writing ability was tested, "All the facts were correctly reproduced, but the composition was poor and the spelling incredibly bad for a highly educated Staff Officer."[29]

Despite this individuation of experimental procedure, Head hoped that the investigative technologies set out in his publications would provide a set of tools which other neurologists could take up and apply in their own studies. He therefore outlined in some detail his procedures along with the conditions under which these tests should be conducted. The patient was to be

> examined alone, in a quiet room, apart from all distracting sights and sounds. It is of fundamental importance to record not only what he says or does, but also every remark or question of the observer. As soon as it is certain that the patient understands the task he is asked to perform, each series of tests must be carried out in silence; should this rule be broken, each side of the conversation must be recorded. It is particularly important to write down at the moment any statement which throws light on the ideas or feelings of the patient with regard to the test, or to the difficulties he experiences in carrying it out.[30]

Such formal protocols could not, however, contain the full range of aptitudes and sensitivities that Head used to achieve his results. Some of his unformulated procedures and unarticulated skills do, however, emerge in the asides that often accompany the more rigidly regimented part of the text.

The tests themselves were designed to scrutinize all aspects of the patient's capacity to employ and comprehend symbols. These examinations

---

[27] Ibid., p. 162.
[28] Ibid., p. 233.
[29] Ibid., p. 247.
[30] Ibid., p. 147.

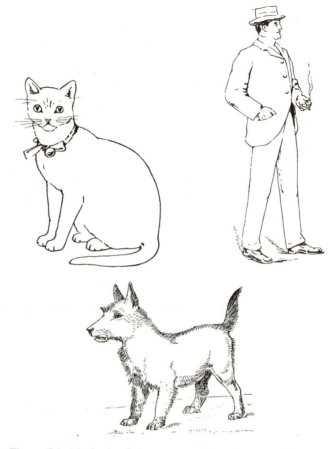

Figure 5.1. Methods of examination, "Reading from Pictures."
Henry Head, *Aphasia and Kindred Disorders of Speech* (1926)

were arranged in a continuum of difficulty. Among the simpler tests were those in which the patient's ability to recognize and name objects was tested in a variety of ways. The results were then recorded in tabular form. The "man, cat and dog test" was, in Head's words, designed "to investigate the power of reading and writing in its simplest and most elementary form."[31] The patient was asked to "read" from a series of pictures shown to him in various combinations; it is instructive to remark what *kind* of man is represented (fig. 5.1).

Some of the more demanding of the tests illustrate the unusually extensive notion of symbolic function with which Head operated. For instance,

---

[31] Ibid., p. 153.

he would show his patients two clock faces marked in arabic numerals (as, he notes, were most wristwatches used during the war) and then ask them to set and tell the time under various conditions. Some of the operations these tests demanded were not trials of language as such but of the patient's capacity for symbolic comprehension more generally. They were, in particular, a test of the patient's ability to grasp the *meaning* inherent in the relations between the numerals on the clock face and the two hands.

The "hand, eye and ear tests" at first glance appear to be still more remote from an investigation of linguistic capacity. The patient was seated opposite the observer and asked to mimic his movements. Head noted that this was one of the instances in which it was necessary to be acquainted with an individual's prior abilities before one could arrive at any conclusions on his current functional deficits. Some normal people, he remarked, had difficulty in performing an extended series of these imitative movements; others, however, "can carry them out perfectly, especially if they are young and intelligent, and belong to the class from which so many of my war patients were drawn."[32]

But why was the ability to perform such imitative movements deemed relevant to the assessment of aphasic patients? Head noted that when an individual failed to imitate correctly the movement of someone in front of him, he might succeed in copying the same movement seen in a mirror. Head explained this difference by claiming that an unarticulated verbal element intervened in the first case between the patient seeing the observer's movement and his then seeking to imitate it; in particular, when face to face the patient was obliged to make a distinction between the left and right sides of his body and those of the observer, and this discrimination required some internal verbalization. Characteristically, Head cited a patient's own explanation of this phenomenon: "Your sitting opposite to me, that helps make the thing a bit mystery. Say to myself, then it's gone again; I lost it, don't hold it long enough."[33] In the case of movements observed in the mirror, such translation was not required; imitation was merely "automatic."

There were also a number of tests which scrutinized what might be called collateral functions. Head asked his patients to make groundplans of the rooms they occupied in order to ascertain their appreciation of spatial relations. They were also required to draw pictures. Head followed Pierre Marie's lead in choosing an elephant as the subject of these drawings. This test was supposed to provide an insight into the state of a patient's visual imagery and into his ability to translate that imagery into an accurate composition.

[32] Ibid., p. 157.
[33] Ibid., p. 282.

The information derived from these tests was compiled into a series of tables which formed an important feature of Head's text. But as well as the tabulated results of these investigations, Head allowed space for his select patients' own representation of their condition. To an extent, they were allowed to be the authors of their own histories. Head frequently quoted the patient's own understanding of his condition with little or no gloss as an authentic depiction of his pathology. For example, Pierre Marie's notion of a "pure anarthria" was invalidated by quoting the words of a patient suffering from what at first glance might appear an uncomplicated "motor aphasia."[34]

Another "highly intelligent officer" was also allowed his say while Head confined his editorial activity to pointing out the faults of pronunciation to which this patient was subject:

> I'm confine (confined) to the words I've got back since my speech came back. I try to make a statement—I have to use the words I've got back—when they say, "What do you mean by so and so?" I haven't got a further example of what I've said, to explain. My vocabulary (pronounced "vocab-lery") is still small. When I try to explain I haven't got the words I want, and when they say over a set of words, I then say "Yes, that's the one." I have to go over the roots; I trace the root back to the Latin, or that, and get it eventually (pronounced "e-venchaly").[35]

This was a narrative of the lived experience of being deprived of the full exercise of language; but it was an account that was nonetheless allowed an epistemological status equal to that of the physician. Indeed, on occasion an "intelligent patient" was held to have arrived independently at some significant insight about the nature of his condition.[36] The patient was permitted to *explain* the nature of his own symptoms, and Head was prepared to accept such explanations—even when, due to the nature of the affliction, these accounts came out "somewhat rambling."[37] Head might even in the light of a patient's self-exegesis be led to modify his investigative strategy.[38]

When words failed completely, pantomime might still allow the subject to perform this heuristic function.[39] Head emphasized the varied and ingenious stratagems to which patients would resort to overcome the obstacles that their conditions placed in the way of their acting as Head's collocutors. One patient "managed to indicate his likes, dislikes and desires by

---

[34] Head, "Aphasia," p. 113.
[35] Ibid., p. 114.
[36] Head, *Aphasia*, vol. 1, p. 244.
[37] Ibid., p. 191.
[38] Ibid., p. 195.
[39] Ibid., p. 171; see also p. 182.

the combination of his scanty vocabulary with expressive gestures. . . . Thus, I was able to elicit from him much more information than would have seemed possible from the few words he possessed for voluntary use." He was, for instance,

> able to tell me how he had acquired the power of imitating correctly my move-ments in the hand, eye and ear tests, which at first puzzled him considerably. He wanted to explain that, as soon as he discovered he must make an appar-ently opposite movement, the task became easy. He thrust one hand forwards and simultaneously drew the other backwards exclaiming, "I got to go . . . see?"; then he said, "See . . . goes, you know," and made similar movements in the reverse direction.[40]

Such insistence upon communicative competence is eloquent testimony to the importance that Head attached to validating the patient's status as conversational partner and experimental collaborator in his text. But this passage is evidence also of the enthusiasm with which his "subjects" en-gaged with this ambiguous and demanding role. It is tempting to specu-late that for these individuals this activity served a therapeutic purpose; it may be that Head's text betrays evidence of more than one agenda.

The Varieties of Aphasia

On the basis of tests of these kinds carried out over a period of several years on a group of around twenty-six select patients, Head declared it was possible to identify "the empirical groups of aphasia and kindred dis-orders of speech produced by an organic cerebral lesion."[41] He held that it was possible to distinguish four such categories, although he emphasized that all such classifications of language disorders were necessarily crude and arbitrary; as a holist, he was committed to the view that there were no sharp divisions in nature itself. Nonetheless, Head insisted that his groups were "empirical," the result of letting the phenomena speak for themselves, in contrast to the arbitrarily imposed classifications of earlier aphasiology.

Head called the first of his empirical groups "verbal defects." They were primarily characterized by defective word formation. The second category was that of "syntactical defects": in these cases the patient had no lack of words, but spoke a kind of nonsensical jargon. In the third group of "nom-inal defects" the patient had difficulty in naming objects correctly.

---

[40] Ibid., p. 171.
[41] Ibid., p. 220.

The fourth grouping—"semantic defects"—is perhaps the most revealing of Head's general orientation to language and its disorders. It reflects his basic notion of the human organism as an active, adaptive agent rather than a mechanism subject to various predictable defects. In defects of this sort the patient had difficulty in grasping the meaning of propositions and conversely of himself formulating and executing meaningful verbal operations. Head contrasted this notion of the linguistic subject and his disorders with the more passive conceptions of earlier students of aphasia. He claimed, for instance, that certain aphasics' inability to perform imitative actions

> are entirely inexplicable on any theory of "motor" and "sensory" aphasia, "apraxia" and "agnosia," or similar analytical conceptions; but they fall into place at once if we assume that the main defect consisted in loss of power to evoke verbal symbols at will and to formulate them with a view to action.[42]

The figure of the healthy subject as one possessing the *power* to manipulate symbols in a purposeful fashion is one that recurs in Head's text. The converse of this concept is a vision of the aphasic as powerless and passive: a feminized victim of the sort found in John Hughlings Jackson's writings. But it is notable that Head's aphasics tend not to be entirely supine and hapless; they retain a degree of control over the symbols they once commanded. The prior "person" is not entirely subsumed by the pathology, but struggles for expression against the novel constraints imposed upon him. "Every case of aphasia," Head maintained, "is the response of an individual to some want of power to employ language and represents a personal reaction to mechanical difficulties in speech."[43] It is this residual competence and capacity for resistance that enabled these patients to play so active a role in Head's investigative enterprise.

Constructing Pathology

Having arrived at a set of reasonably coherent clinical syndromes, Head now confronted the task of establishing with injury to which part of the brain these symptoms were regularly associated. His strictures upon nineteenth-century notions of localization have already been noted; he nonetheless maintained that: "No one doubts that speech in its highest forms can be disturbed by destruction of the tissues of the brain, or that the

---

[42] Ibid., p. 204.
[43] Ibid., p. 289.

manifestations differ according to the situation of the lesion."[44] Even an avowed iconoclast was unable to dispense entirely with the constraints of the organicist discourse.

But when it came to determining the situation of the lesions corresponding to Head's four clinical categories, a problem arose. As we have seen, the soldier-patients upon whom Head had based his theories were admirably suited to the purposes of clinical investigation. However, the very qualities that made them such good subjects of scientific inquiry—their youth and general good health—also had another, less convenient, corollary: they were unlikely to succumb to their injuries and thus become available for autopsy within the period of the investigation.

How then was Head to ascertain which parts of their brain had been damaged by the bullet or other missile? Head made elaborate efforts to solve this problem—for instance by making careful diagrams of the entry and exit wounds on the surface of the head. He also took radiograms of different aspects of the head in all of his cases. By these means it was possible to reach certain general conclusions about the areas of the brain affected in each instance. Moreover, when surgery was undertaken on one of these patients, Head ensured that he was present to record "any indications that could be used for cerebral localisation." He noted that: "Such autopsies in the living often furnish evidence of the greatest value,"[45] a revealing understanding of surgical intervention.

Head also sought, however, a technology that would create a closer analogue to the direct examination of a patient's brain that was normally available only after death. He tried to attain this by a method that might be called "autopsy by proxy." The invention of this technology required the cooperation of another set of allies: namely, Grafton Elliot Smith, the Professor of Anatomy at University College London, and various of his colleagues at the Anatomical Institute—and, one might add, of the cadavers deposited within that establishment.

Head had begun to collaborate with Elliot Smith before the latter took up his post at University College. In his paper on "Sensation and the Cerebral Cortex" published in 1918, Head had faced a similar problem to that presented in his researches on aphasia: namely, "It is impossible to determine with accuracy the position of the injury to the brain from the situation of the wound on the surface." But it was possible to arrive at some rough conclusions: "and Professor Elliot Smith has kindly attempted to localise the main incidence of the lesion in each of my cases."[46] Here Elliot

---

[44] Ibid., p. 431.
[45] Ibid., p. 443.
[46] Head, *Studies*, vol. 2, pp. 789–790.

Smith's contribution lay purely in his acknowledged expertise in the topography of the cerebral convolutions; from an examination of the wounds he plotted the likely position of the underlying injury on a standardized map of the cortex.

But it was after his appointment to the Chair of Anatomy at University College in 1919 that Elliot Smith was to be of most service to Head. The relationship was reciprocal inasmuch as the kind of demands that Head made of the Anatomical Institute were in keeping with Elliot Smith's disciplinary goals. Upon acceding to the Chair at University College he took upon himself the task of attempting to revitalize anatomy as an academic discipline and to acquire for it a renewed status among the medical and biological sciences. He approached this task largely by forging alliances with other disciplines, such as anthropology and psychology, with which anatomy could enjoy a mutually beneficial engagement. Elliot Smith maintained, in particular, that "anatomical work in neurology is enormously helped by association with Clinical Neurology, and what we have been trying to build up here is a neurological section in this Institute in which the strictly morphological work is combined with experimental work as well as clinical investigation."

Writing in 1925 he noted that "The sort of clinical work that Dr. Henry Head has been doing is obviously of the utmost importance both to physical and cultural anthropology."[47] Elliot Smith had in fact used Head's investigations on aphasia in his own attempts to construct an evolutionary history of human brain function. He constructed a narrative in which brain development was the motor of progress in human evolution; in Landau's words, "The critical events and 'struggles' go on . . . in the skull-vault or brain-chamber."[48] More particularly, Elliot Smith equated human evolutionary progress with "a steady growth and specialization of certain parts of the brain."[49] The final transformation from ape to man occurred when, at the appropriate moment, this brain acquired the capacity to name objects and to think symbolically.[50]

When he came to chart the stages of the process whereby man acquired his linguistic capacities, Elliot Smith relied heavily upon Head's categori-

---

[47] Warren R. Dawson, *Sir Grafton Elliot Smith: A Biographical Record by His Colleagues* (London: Jonathan Cape, 1938), p. 92.

[48] Misia Landau, *Narratives of Human Evolution* (New Haven: Yale University Press, 1991), p. 109.

[49] G. Elliot Smith, *The Evolution of Man: Essays* (London: Oxford University Press, 1924), p. 45.

[50] Landau, *Narratives*, pp. 125–127. For a more conventional view of Elliot Smith's place in the history of physical anthropology see: Peter J. Bowler, *Theories of Human Evolution: A Century of Debate, 1844–1944* (Baltimore: Johns Hopkins University Press, 1986), pp. 167–173.

zation of the different forms of aphasia. At an early juncture, *names* were invented; this point in evolution corresponded to Head's class of "nominal" disorders. "But," Elliot Smith insisted,

> it required a much more elaborate cultivation of the acoustic territories of the cortex before real sentences were devised by the syntactic process of linking together a series of words to express a meaning which was not simply that of the individual words or the combination of them, but, so to speak, a glorified word with an individuality and a meaning of its own and a rhythm of enunciation somewhat akin to music.

A disruption of this process through injury to the cortex gave rise to what Head had called "syntactic" defects. As a complement of the evolution of syntactic ability, there came "a wider understanding of the significance of the symbolism so elaborated"—the physiological corollary of Head's "semantic" dysfunctions.[51]

The benefit that Head in turn derived from his alliance with Elliot Smith took the form of access to material resources and technical aptitudes rather than a borrowing of theoretical tools. He made use of the skills and materials available at the Anatomical Institute to create a kind of surrogate cadaver to take the place of his still living patients. Drawing upon the supply of bodies available in the Institute, he and his associates selected ones in which the head was as close as possible of the same dimensions as that of the individual whose wound was to be localized. The exact size of the external wound was marked out on the scalp and holes drilled through the skull to mark its dimensions:

> Through these a coloured fluid was passed with a small brush to fix the relation of the bony opening to the surface of the brain. Then the skull-cap was removed and a cast taken of its inner surface. This gave us a solid representation of the brain, covered by its membranes, on which were indicated the limits of the external wound.[52]

The contours of the cadaver's brain were then determined by means of a careful dissection and the principal features drawn on the cast: "Thus we finally obtained a record of the area occupied by the wound on the surface of the brain, together with its extent in relation to the main landmarks of cerebral topography."[53] Photographs of the end product of these labors were included in *Aphasia and Kindred Disorders of Speech* (fig. 5.2).

[51] Elliot Smith, *Evolution*, p. 153.
[52] Head, *Aphasia*, vol. 1, pp. 443–444.
[53] Ibid., p. 444.

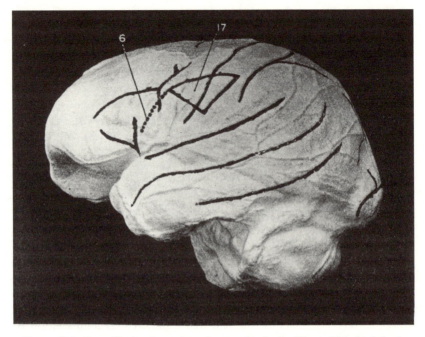

Figure 5.2. Site of lesion in various forms of aphasia. Henry Head, *Aphasia and Kindred Disorders of Speech* (1926)

The result of these operations was the creation of a three-dimensional map on which regular correlations between symptoms and site of lesion could be plotted. Although the technology was more elaborate, the object of the exercise was closer than Head might have admitted to the goals of the "old" aphasiology. His emphasis on the need for the most painstaking *precision* in making these maps was, however, distinctive; it was expressive of a particular notion of scientific virtue.

By means of these techniques Head believed that he had attained the second half of his program. He had found a means of associating the syndromes he had isolated through his clinical investigations with injuries to determinate parts of the brain. His mastery over the condition was now complete. "Verbal" aphasia, Head concluded, was associated with a lesion situated in the lower portion of the central convolutions or in their underlying structures. In cases of "syntactical" aphasia it was possible to be equally confident and assert that this form of language disorder arose when the temporal lobes were injured. Head felt that the material at his disposal obliged him to be less dogmatic about the localization of his other two categories. Nonetheless, there was, he held, little doubt that nominal and semantic aphasia were the result of injuries located between the post-central fissure and the occipital lobe.

Conclusion

Head presented his work on aphasia as marking an important new departure in the history of the field. As we have seen, he cast doubt on the value of most of what had previously been written on the subject. The experience of war encouraged him, as it did so many of his contemporaries, to represent his era as one of cataclysmic change in which old ways of thinking were being overthrown and replaced by radically different systems. Head's writings were a self-conscious harbinger of a new, fundamentally different, neurology. Within them he played the part of the iconoclast who put commitment to empirical inquiry above devotion to received dogma.

Some of Head's colleagues agreed with this assessment of Head's heroic role in the history of neurology. James Collier, in a discussion of Head's views held at the Royal Society of Medicine in November 1920, pointed to a "growing revolution against the former conceptions of the nature of the speech function and the explanation of its defects," which had culminated in "Dr Head's bold endeavour to place this subject upon a sounder and truer foundation."[54] Others, however, were less convinced that this was a true revolution. They tempered the progressive fervor of Head's admirers with a conservative skepticism. For instance, Sir James Purves Stewart, who had himself undertaken extensive investigations upon soldiers with head wounds, maintained that Head's clinical groupings were merely an unnecessary invocation of new terminology to describe syndromes with which neurologists were already familiar.[55]

But if we consider the literature of aphasia *as* a body of literature, there is no doubt that Head's case histories do represent a departure from the predominant nineteenth-century form of clinical narrative. The essence of this difference lies in the relationship between patient and doctor, subject and observer, that these documents embody. I have already hinted at the element of collegiality present in the interaction between Head and certain of his patients—those whom he considered his "best" experimental subjects.[56] This status of partnership is quite different from that found in the typical nineteenth-century aphasic case history in which the patient has the status of a reified object of the clinical gaze.

In Head's optimal case histories, on the other hand, the gaze has become internalized; the patient is his own observer seeking, in collabora-

---

[54] "Discussion," p. 413.

[55] Ibid., pp. 424–432.

[56] In his obituary of his former colleague, George Riddoch noted the importance of Head's own "personality" in attracting "intelligent patients into his fold; they could not resist the glamour and excitement of his work on themselves, and became ardent collaborators." *London Times*, 18 October 1940.

tion with his physician, to arrive at a shared understanding of his afflic-tion.[57] The conversational mode accordingly occupies a novel prominence in these narratives. The linguistic disabilities of these individuals notwith-standing, Head insisted on their ability to act as competent interlocutors.[58] As well as what is ascertained by the formal regime of tests, Head and his associates therefore learn a great deal by simply engaging in ordinary social intercourse with the wounded officers in their charge. One of these pa-tients, "Captain C.," was, Head recalled, "a charming companion."[59]

One illustration will suffice. To prove that patients suffering from "syn-tactical" aphasia retained a high degree of intelligence despite the appar-ently nonsensical nature of their utterances, Head recounted the following anecdote. Major X, a patient showing the signs of this form of speech disorder,

> was walking in Kew Gardens with the medical officer in charge of the hospital, when he pointed out a new variety of heath. The doctor said "Scotch," to which the patient replied, "No, no, you and me." It was a rare Irish heath, and both the patient and his companion were Irishmen.[60]

Head's readiness to treat his patients as equals—as colleagues rather than mere subjects—thus had a great influence upon the form and content of his case histories. It is, however, important to note that the mode of gentlemanly conversation[61] forms only one element in the overall texture of his narratives. Some of his patients were indeed allowed the status of concrete individuals, endowed with a distinct "personality" that helped to establish the character of their complaint, and with an "intelligence" that qualified them as competent collaborators. But at the same time these patients mattered because they possessed an exemplary value. Where

[57] Head does not cite any sources for his style of investigation; his overriding claims to originality perhaps militated against any such acknowledgments. But it is worth noting that his style of "collegial" inquiry bears a stronger resemblance to German forms of academic psychological investigation than it does to more strictly clinical examinations; crucial to the distinction is the relative power of subject and experimenter in the two types of scientific work. On this contrast see: Kurt Danziger, *Constructing the Subject: Historical Origins of Psychological Research* (Cambridge: Cambridge University Press, 1990), pp. 49–63.

[58] Conversely, former patients waxed lyrical about Head's own range and skill as a conver-sationalist: Robert Nichols, *London Times*, 15 October 1940.

[59] Head, *Aphasia*, vol. 1, p. 256.

[60] Ibid., p. 239.

[61] For a strong claim about the role of "civil conversation" in the genealogy of the scien-tific method see: Steven Shapin, *A Social History of Truth: Civility and Science in Seventeenth-Century England* (Chicago: University of Chicago Press, 1994), especially pp. 119–125. It is necessary to distinguish, as Head himself did, between gentlemanly conversation and "the conversation I reserve for my servant." Letter to Ruth Mayhew, 14 July 1901 [?], CMAC, PP HEA D4/9.

Head's schema was supposed to differ from those of his predecessors was that it arose from a faithful rendering of the facts of each case; it was not brutally imposed upon a recalcitrant clinical material.

Head could scarcely contain his enthusiasm when he referred to them variously as "splendid" or "superb" examples of the particular clinical forms he was trying to establish.[62] He had in 1901 reflected upon the apparent perversity of applying such positive terms to cases of disease. "When dealing with natural knowledge," he wrote, "things that are true need not be beautiful and when I say 'what a beautiful case' I mean that it exemplifies some truth though it may be in itself foul."[63] One is reminded of the paradoxical complicity that Derrida sees between "clinical" and "critical" commentary:

> At the moment when criticism ... allegedly protects the meaning of a thought or the value of a work against psychomedical reductions, it comes to the same result through the opposite path: *it creates an example*. That is to say, *a case*. A work or an adventure of thought is made to bear witness, as example or martyr, to a structure whose essential permanence becomes the prime preoccupation of the commentary.[64]

Head allowed his patients a voice only in order to spirit it away in order to elucidate an essential natural order.[65]

When in this mode, the personality of these individuals recedes into the background; what matters is their status as ciphers for certain types of pathology. Their personal attributes are ultimately significant because they provide an especially pellucid medium in which the disorder can expose itself. At the dénouement of these narratives, the protagonist ceases to be a person and becomes *the* brain—there can of course only be one brain, hence the plausibility of an autopsy by proxy.

Despite their aspirations to a revolutionary status, Head's texts are impregnated by social conservatism. Certain aspects of his case histories can be read as yet another literary illustration of the pervasiveness of class distinctions in early twentieth-century British culture. As George Orwell observed, "In 1910, every human being in these islands could be 'placed'

[62] Head, *Aphasia*, vol. 1, p. 446.

[63] Letter to Ruth Mayhew, 5 June 1901, CMAC, D4/8. Head continued that in art, on the other hand, "Beauty and Truth become one."

[64] Jacques Derrida, "La Parole Soufflée," in *Writing and Difference*, trans. Alan Bass (London: Routledge, 1993), pp. 169–195, on p. 170.

[65] As Head remarked in a course of lectures in 1912: "cases of disease will be considered simply as the means by which certain laws are demonstrated & certain physiological activities are laid bare." "Page-May Memorial Lectures on the Afferent Nervous System at Institute of Physiology University College London," CMAC, PP HEA B13.

in an instant by his clothes, manners and accent."[66] Even sickness and injury could not erase these distinctions in the clinic.[67] Given the prominence of speech as a marker of class difference, it is unsurprising that affections of language should prove a site at which awareness of class became particularly manifest.[68] The social status ascribed to the officer-patient, in part at least because of his linguistic identity, made him more intelligible than a private soldier both to himself and to the investigator. Anatomy, however, proved to be a great leveller.

Head's texts therefore display a disjunction. At the level of the clinical they deal with embodied subjects, concrete individuals who themselves help to shape their own case history. The durable integrity of these personalities is signified by the *resistance* to disease that they display and the ingenuity with which they circumvent the disabilities imposed upon them. But when Head turns to pathology proper this particularity is lost; sensitivity to the individual is subsumed by the will to a universal truth. With the delegated autopsy the patient ceases to be an agent and becomes an effect of pathology. Even an avowed rebel ultimately succumbed to the authority of disciplinary morality.

[66] Quoted in Fussell, *The Great War*, p. 197.

[67] In a somewhat analogous move Head's former collaborator W. H. R. Rivers had distinguished between the forms of war neurosis appropriate to "officer and man"; in this instance, the greater complexity of the mental life of the former ensured that he reacted to the stresses of combat in a more refined and nuanced way. *Instinct and the Unconscious: A Contribution to a Biological Theory of the Psycho-Neuroses*, 2nd ed. (Cambridge: Cambridge University Press, 1922), p. 209. For a fuller discussion see: Elaine Showalter, *The Female Malady: Women, Madness and English Culture, 1830–1980* (London: Virago, 1987), pp. 174–175.

[68] On language as an indicator of social boundaries see: Patrick Joyce, *Visions of the People: Industrial England and the Question of Class 1848–1914* (Cambridge: Cambridge University Press, 1991), p. 157.

SIX

DISSONANT VOICES

CHAPTER THREE provided an account of the "discourse" of aphasia. The concept was intended to reconcile two apparently contradictory aspects of the way in which a body of knowledge about the new disease was created and maintained. Discourse in this instance does not denote a preexistent framework that determined the forms of scientific creativity characteristic of the period. The discourse was constituted, maintained, and renewed by the constant activity and work of those engaged in this field of scientific endeavor. On the other hand, this endeavor was only possible because of a certain lack of freedom: it depended upon the constraint acting upon those involved in the processes of creation, dissemination, and replication.

The notion of a language game might appear to capture this tense duality at least as well. A game involves both a free play of elements and a framework within which that liberty is exercised; without these rules there would be no meaning or coherence to the actions of the players.[1] The notion of a language game is, however, ultimately overrestrictive. The making and maintenance of aphasia did not involve merely a set of symbolic exchanges, although the generation of texts was central to the process. Aphasiology occurred in real clinical and pedagogic spaces permeated by relations of power.[2] Moreover, the virtual space of textual exchange was no less hierarchical and asymmetrical in nature. While the alternative formulation "a form of life" is less objectionable, only the Foucauldian concept of discourse does full justice to this power/knowledge nexus.

---

[1] For an application of the notion of a language game to the historical understanding of science see: Steven Shapin and Simon Schaffer, *Leviathan and the Air-Pump: Hobbes, Boyle, and the Experimental Method* (Princeton: Princeton University Press, 1985), pp. 14–15. Compare Derrida's formulation: "the writer writes *in* a language and *in* a logic whose proper system, laws, and life his discourse by definition cannot dominate absolutely. He uses them only by letting himself, after a fashion and up to a point, be governed by the system." Jacques Derrida, *Of Grammatology*, trans. Gaytari Chakravorty Spivak, (Baltimore: Johns Hopkins Press, 1974), p. 158. While this passage does express the necessary dialectic between constraint and individual creativity, it does, of course, beg the question of after *what* fashion and to *which* point the writer "lets" himself be used.

[2] Richard Terdiman, *Discourse/Counter-Discourse: The Theory of Symbolic Resistance in Nineteenth-Century France* (Ithaca: Cornell University Press, 1990), p. 56.

Apart from necessary asymmetries of power in its fine texture,[3] a discourse is authoritarian inasmuch as it is necessarily exclusive. It endows a particular set of representations with the status of truth; other representations are actively repressed or, if the discourse is secure, forgotten. But this selectivity in reception and recognition does not imply that the discourse is necessarily monolithic and characterized by consensus. We have seen that controversy was essential to the practice of aphasiology—as evinced, for instance, in the competition between different schemata each purporting to give a more adequate mapping of the sites and locations of the language centers of the brain.

Such disputes did not, however, challenge the overall coherence of the discourse. On the contrary, such differences over detail were productive rather than destructive; they made work for the community of practitioners. They can be seen as the stuff of normal science. Practitioners who raised more fundamental doubts about the validity of the ruling metaphors—such as the French neurologist Charles-Édouard Brown Séquard (1817–94)—were marginal, scarcely audible, figures.[4]

But, according to a long established narrative, around the turn of the twentieth century a more far-reaching and destabilizing dissent became vocal. Some of this criticism came from outside the medical-scientific community. As early as 1881 the linguist Heymann Steinthal, asserted that, putting to one side the continuing disputes about the location of the various language centers, "the entire approach to the question [*Betrachtungsweise*] appears inadequate to me." This inadequacy derived in large part from the character of the typical aphasiological case history, which Steinthal deemed to be "incomplete and inexact." Above all, this genre of writing tended to neglect the *psychic* side of the case.[5] Although he viewed the classic aphasia literature from an entirely different perspective,

---

[3] "The seigneurial privilege of giving names even allows us to conceive of the origin of language itself as a manifestation of the power of the rulers: they say 'this is so and so', they set their seal on everything and every occurrence with a sound and thereby take possession of it, as it were." Friedrich Nietzsche, *On the Genealogy of Morality*, ed. Keith Ansell-Pearson (Cambridge: Cambridge University Press, 1994), p. 13.

[4] Brown-Séquard rejected the dominant model of cortical "seats" for the language functions. He argued that language loss consequent upon cortical injury should instead be understood as a reflex phenomenon. See: P. J. Koehler, "Brown-Séquard and Cerebral Localization as Illustrated by his Ideas on Aphasia," *Journal of the History of the Neurosciences* 5 (1996): 26–33. For an early statement of Brown-Séquard's views on aphasia see: "On the Importance of the Application of Physiology to the Practice of Medicine and Surgery," *Dublin Quarterly Journal of Medical Science* 39ns (1865): 421–436, p. 429.

[5] Heymann Steinthal, *Einleitung in die Psychologie und Sprachwissenschaft* (Berlin: Ferd. Dümmlers, 1881), pp. 463–464. See: Paul Eling, "Steinthal's Psycholinguistic Interpretation of Language Disorders," in H. Grundlach (ed.), *Arbeiten zur Psychologie Geschichte* (Göttingen: Hogrefe, 1994), pp. 177–88.

Steinthal's strictures thus strongly resembled those seen in the work of John Hughlings Jackson and Henry Head (see chapters 4 and 5).

Similar misgivings came eventually to have currency within the medical literature itself. The unquestioned premises of classical aphasia studies were challenged and alternative, previously suppressed, ways of under-standing language loss articulated. This disruptive movement is usually referred to as part of the "holistic reaction" to the mechanistic models of mind and brain function favored in the nineteenth century; and contem-poraries acknowledged it as a tendency that challenged some of the funda-mental tenets prevalent since the 1860s.[6] The discourse had lost perhaps the greatest guarantee of its dominance: its invisiblity. Thus, writing in 1910, Maurice Brissot remarked that recently the "dogma created by Broca and his pupils" had been subjected to the most radical criticism and challenged by putatively superior principles.[7]

Brissot referred in particular to the writings of the Parisian neurologist, Pierre Marie (1853–1940). As a young doctor Marie had been a protege of Charcot, a fact to which he alluded in his work. He wrote on numerous neurological topics including diseases of the spinal cord as well as publish-ing contributions to general medicine. After 1897, however, when he joined the staff of the Bicêtre Hospital in Paris, he became preoccupied with the subject of aphasia. Of all those who challenged neurological or-thodoxy in the early years of the twentieth century, Marie was the most self-consciously revolutionary: among the epithets that his efforts earned him were "Marie the Iconoclast" and Marie the "destroyer and re-former."[8] Marie's works therefore provide a locus classicus for a study of the strategies of subversion that were deployed against the edifice of classi-cal aphasiology, and much of this chapter will be devoted to their analysis.

Marie's work is regarded as symptomatic of a more general reaction against the certainties of nineteenth-century brain science with all the ideological load that it carried.[9] Two other texts often considered as repre-

[6] See: Anne Harrington, "A Feeling for the 'Whole': The Holistic Reaction in Neurology from the *Fin de Siècle* to the Interwar Years," in Mikulas Teich and Roy Porter (eds.), *Fin de Siècle and its Legacy* (Cambridge: Cambridge University Press, 1990), pp. 254–277. For a contemporary review see: James Collier, "Recent Work on Aphasia," *Brain* 31 (1908): 521–549.

[7] Maurice Brissot, *L'aphasie dans ses rapports avec la dèmence et les vésanies. (Étude histo-rique, clinique et diagnostique considérations médico-légales)* (Paris: G. Steintheil, 1910), p. 7.

[8] Henry Head, *Aphasia and Kindred Disorders of Speech*, 2 vols. (Cambridge: Cambridge University Press, 1926), vol. 1, p. 67; Collier, "Recent Work," p. 527.

[9] The best source for the wider reaction to positivism in the late nineteenth and early twentieth century remains: H. Stuart Hughes, *Consciousness and Society: The Reorientation of European Thought 1890–1930* (St Albans: Granada, 1974). See also the essays in: Dorothy Ross (ed.), *Modernist Impulses in the Human Sciences 1870–1930* (Baltimore: Johns Hopkins Press, 1994).

sentative of this movement will also be considered. One, written by a neurologist, may be viewed as internal to the discourse: a technical revision of certain aspects of classical aphasiology, the implications of which could, however, be read as challenges of a more fundamental kind. The other text, written by a philosopher, viewed the science of aphasia from the outside; it sought to undermine its certainties because of their perceived place in a larger, inimical cultural configuration. I will in particular be concerned with the devices and strategies by which these texts destabilize the certainties of classical aphasia studies. Of special prominence is their questioning of metaphor and their manipulation of narrative.

Freud's *Zur Auffassung der Aphasien*

In 1891 Sigmund Freud (1856–1939) published a short monograph dedicated to interpreting the various forms of aphasia.[10] Freud had trained in medicine at the University of Vienna and developed a special interest in diseases of the nervous system; he spent four months in Paris studying under Charcot. After his return to Vienna Freud was invited to contribute an article on aphasia to a medical encyclopaedia. His subsequent book endeavored to present a novel view of the subject.

Freud's introduction observed the conventions of academic modesty by acknowledging the contributions to this field made by "some of the best brains of German and foreign neurology,"[11] and by setting for himself apparently circumscribed goals. The conception of aphasia developed by his predecessors contained, Freud alleged, "two assumptions which might profitably be revised." Ostensibly therefore Freud is no revolutionary; he purports to do no more than modify aspects of the existing structure of aphasiology. His is to be a "contribution" to a ruling discourse not a challenge to its authority.

---

[10] For a discussion of this work in the context of Freud's other writings see: John C. Marshall, "Freud's Psychology of Language," in Richard Wollheim (ed.), *Freud: A Collection of Critical Essays* (New York: Doubleday, 1974), 349–365. Freud's work on aphasia has drawn attention chiefly because of its supposed foreshadowing of certain aspects of his later psychoanalytic writing, such as verbal slips; see, for example: John Forrester, *Language and the Origins of Psychoanalysis* (London: Macmillan, 1980), pp. 14–29.

[11] Sigmund Freud, *On Aphasia: A Critical Study*, trans. E. Stengel (London: Imago, 1953), p. 1 [1]. Figures in brackets are references to the corresponding passage in the original: *Zur Auffassung des Aphasien: Eine kritische Studie* (Leipzig: Franz Deuticke, 1891). Freud's private remarks subvert his public modesty; he wrote to Wilhelm Fliess on 2 May 1891 that in this book: "I am very impudent, cross swords with your friend Wernicke, with Lichtheim and Grashey, and even scratch the high and mighty idol Meynert." Jeffrey Moussaieff Masson (ed.), *The Complete Letters of Sigmund Freud to Wilhelm Fliess* (Cambridge, Mass.: Belknap Press, 1985), p. 28. I refrain from any Oedipal reading of the passage.

The first of the two assumptions Freud saw as a candidate for revision was suitably technical. A tendency had arisen especially since the publication of Ludwig Lichtheim's paper of 1885[12] to differentiate between aphasias attributable to lesions of the language "centers" of the brain and others to be ascribed to the commissures supposed to communicate between them. The other assumption was also apparently abstruse: namely, the views first sketched by Carl Wernicke and later taken up by others of the topographic relations between the various cortical language centers.

But at the outset of his discussion Freud hinted at the peculiar strategic significance of these two foci. They were "intimately related to the idea of 'localization', i.e. of the restriction of nervous functions to anatomically definable areas, which pervades the whole of recent neuropathology."[13] Any tinkering with these two topics had therefore the potential to translate into a reappraisal of one of the primary goals of the entire aphasiological project. Freud could therefore with some plausibility be depicted as a Kepler setting out to simplify the "Ptolemy-like" confusion into which the aphasiological universe had descended.[14]

"For decades," Freud remarked, "we have been endeavoring to advance our knowledge of the localization of functions by the study of clinical symptoms."[15] This endeavor had, in fact, formed the core morality of the discourse of aphasia to which its various technologies, most notably the diagram and the brain map, were subservient. So obvious and natural had this imperative appeared that it was rarely articulated; by now drawing attention to its silent presence at the center of aphasia studies Freud opened up the possibility of a scrutiny of its contingency and of the constraints it had imposed upon the workings of the science.

In particular, Freud drew attention to the role of certain key terms in the execution of the localizationist design. Perhaps the most important of these was "center"—the circumscribed area on the surface of the cortex supposedly endowed with special functional significance:

> under the influence of Meynert's teachings, the theory has been evolved that the speech apparatus consists of distinct cortical centres; their cells are supposed to contain the word images . . . ; these centres are said to be separated by functionless cortical territory, and linked to each other by the association tracts.[16]

[12] L. Lichtheim, "On Aphasia," *Brain* 7 (1885): 433–484.

[13] Freud, *On Aphasia*, p. 1 [1–2].

[14] Ernest Jones, *Sigmund Freud: Life and Work*, 3 vols. (London: Hogarth Press, 1953), vol. 1, p. 235.

[15] Freud, *On Aphasia*, p. 30 [31].

[16] Ibid., p. 54 [56].

The locus classicus for this position was found in the writings of Carl Wernicke.

The centers were, in short, conceived as *depots* in which the elements of language were stored. Anatomical facts and conjectures had been invoked to bolster the credibility of this model. Freud cited Wernicke's claim that: "The cerebral cortex with its 600 millions of cells according to Meynert's estimation, offers a sufficiently great number of storage places in which the innumerable sensory impressions provided by the outer world can be stored one by one without interference."[17] These word dumps were discrete; communication between them depended on the integrity of determinate nervous pathways.

The passage from Wernicke illustrates the altogether prosaic status of this notion of cerebral organization and function. The abundance of cells in the cortex served to prove that the structure of the cortex was equal to the functional role assigned to it. The part played by metaphor in the articulation of the model was effectively suppressed. Yet the notions of depots, storage, and circulation were derived from forms of economic activity; while communication and pathways were equally notions drawn from varieties of human interaction. Cortical space was thus modelled upon particular conceptions of social space; it was a natural economy.

These were in effect dead metaphors: tropes that had by force of usage lost their figurative status. Such blindness to the metaphorical nature of technical language has important consequences for the truth value of models of reality organized around these terms.[18] As Lecercle remarks, "the only metaphors that are alive are the dead ones, as they are the only ones that have been adopted by the community and have survived."[19] In other words, the authority of the "community" ensures that these tropes cease to be regarded as merely, or even at all, metaphorical, but instead enjoy the status of literal descriptions of the material world.

One effect of Freud's text was to revive these defunct but potent metaphors and thereby to challenge the authority vested in them. This action took the form of an explicit strategy in the case of Freud's criticism of Theodor Meynert's account of the structure and operation of the brain. As we have seen, Meynert's writings were often cited as the prime site for authentic and compelling representations of the nature of the brain;

[17] Carl Wernicke, *Der aphasische Symptomencomplex: Eine psychologische Studie auf anatomischer Basis* (Breslau: Max Cohn and Weigert, 1874), p. 5.

[18] For a discussion of the prevalence of various metaphors of brain organization and function in other periods see: John C. Marshall, "Minds, Machines and Metaphors," *Social Studies of Science* 7 (1977): 475–488.

[19] Jean-Jacques Lecercle, *The Violence of Language* (London: Routledge, 1990), p. 161.

Wernicke, for instance, insisted on this point at the outset of his discussion of the phenomena of aphasia.[20]

Freud maintained that Meynert's schema merited the label of "cortico-centric." The cortex was supposedly adapted to the reception and retention of all sensory impressions; from it also emanated motor fibers that allowed it to react to these sensations. He also pointed out that Meynert had sought to impose this model of the nervous system by resort to an explicitly figurative use of language:

> [Meynert] also compared the cerebral cortex to a complex protoplasmic organism which expanded over an object it wanted to incorporate by taking the shape of a cavity. The whole remaining brain thus appeared as an appendix and auxiliary organ of the cerebral cortex, and the whole body as a sheath of feelers and tentacles which enabled it to incorporate and to modify the picture of the external world.[21]

Freud did not directly attack Meynert's master-metaphor for the nervous system, nor did he question the scientific legitimacy of such figurative use of language. But by merely reminding a reader that Meynert's model relied upon a metaphor for at least part of its plausibility he succeeded in casting doubt on its status as a veridical representation of reality. Whatever their virtues, all metaphors are in some respect absurd. In this instance it was easy to imply ways in which the human body was *not* like a jellyfish sheathed in muscle and bone. The figural was, moreover, always vulnerable to stern rebuke from those who assumed the posture of stickler for the unadorned truth: "I wish to draw attention to the fact that the recent advances in the anatomy of the brain have necessitated considerable changes in Meynert's concept of cerebral organization and have thrown doubt on the role attributed by him to the cortex."[22]

Meynert's metaphor was, however, explicit and therefore superficial. Freud's argument also exposed deeper figural elements in current views of the brain. When, in particular, he placed the concept of a "speech center" in inverted commas he rendered visible the metaphoric texture that permeated the discourse of aphasiology; he drew attention to the contingent and arbitrary nature of the linguistic form the science had assumed. "All authors since Wernicke have," he declared,

[20] Wernicke, *Symptomencomplex*, p. 1.

[21] Freud, *On Aphasia*, p. 46 [47–48]. I have slightly modified the translation. Meynert employs this metaphor in several places; for a representative example see: Theodor Meynert, *Psychiatrie. Klinik der Erkrankungen des Vorderhirns begründet auf dessen Bau, Leistungen und Ernährung* (Wien: Wilhelm Braumüller, 1884), pp. 127–128.

[22] Freud, *On Aphasia*, p. 48 [50].

explicitly or implicitly, adopted the view that speech disorders observed clinically, if they have an anatomical basis at all, are caused by lesions of the speech centres or by disruption of the speech association tracts, and that one is therefore justified in differentiating centre aphasias from conduction aphasias.[23]

To the traditional network of centers and commissures Freud applied a version of Occam's razor. He endeavored to show the redundancy of the distinction between aphasias supposedly caused by focal and commissural lesions. Some of the "pathways" depicted by Lichtheim and the like were, moreover, exposed as fictive and equally dispensable entities. Freud also dismissed the notion of language "centers" in which memories serving speech were stored until needed; in Ernest Jones's approving words, he deprived these centers "of their semi-mystical meaning of self-acting agencies."[24]

Freud did not altogether abandon the localizationist imperative. He did, however, demand its revision maintaining that "the speech area is a continuous cortical region within which the associations and transmissions underlying the speech functions are taking place; they are of a complexity beyond comprehension."[25] Freud might have added that it was also beyond *representation*.

The so-called speech centers were no more than the far corners of the speech field. This notion of the cortex as a functional continuum was in marked contrast to the prevailing view of it as partitioned into distinct functional units. Lesions situated near these peripheral zones produced more definite symptoms that those in the interior of the speech region; hence the importance that morbid anatomy had ascribed to such areas as Broca's and Wernicke's region. This special significance, however, "holds only for the pathology, and not for the physiology of the speech apparatus."[26] Aphasiology's ambition to identify the sites responsible for normal function by extrapolation from the evidence of disease was thus cast into doubt. Even from the point of view of the pathology of language, moreover, Freud held that "the significance of the factor of localization has been overrated"; the functional state of the speech apparatus in cases of aphasia was more worthy of attention.[27] An adequate narrative of the brain's workings in disease as in health was at least as significant as any map.

[23] Ibid., p. 10 [10–11].
[24] Jones, *Sigmund Freud*, vol. 1, p. 235.
[25] Freud, *On Aphasia*, p. 62 [64].
[26] Ibid., p. 64 [66].
[27] Ibid., 105 [107].

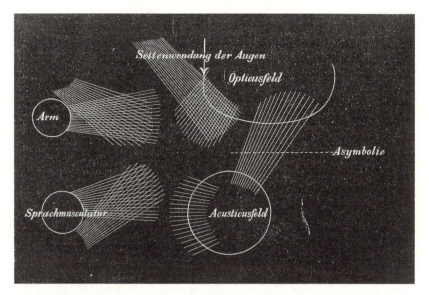

Figure 6.1. Diagram of the "speech association field." Sigmund Freud,
Zur Auffassung der Aphasien (1891)

In common with the exponents of classical aphasiology Freud did adorn his text with a diagram supposed to illustrate the workings of the speech mechanism; much irony, however, attended this gesture.[28] Both in terms of style and import, Freud's figure was quite different from the usual schema. No brain profile was depicted; there were no centers to store the memories of words, and no sign of an "executive" center to control the movements associated with language. Freud's diagram was a minimalist thing of circles representing various "fields" in the cortex with divergent and sometimes intersecting lines indicating commissures between them (fig. 6.1). It was, in effect, a kind of anti-diagram: an implicit rebuke to the elaboration and precision of depiction aspired to by the likes of Lichtheim. This was an admission of obscurity of the subject rather than a celebration of the spectacular power of the gaze.

Freud's text thus exhibits a conception of cortical space at variance with that supposed by classical aphasiology. The latter assumed that each function possessed its preordained niche in the milieu of the brain. The organization of this system lent itself admirably to graphic depiction. The new cortical space was in contrast a far more homogenous yet dynamic entity. Function was diffused; it was, moreover, capable of an active adaptation

[28] Ibid., p. 83.

to changing circumstances. In consequence, its workings varied from time to time. There was an obvious resistance by this brain to any attempt to figure its actions on a two-dimensional surface.[29] The crisis of representation that Freud adumbrated was to become a familiar trope in the neurology of the early twentieth century.

Freud achieved his results to a large extent by problematizing metaphors that were invisible to classical aphasiology. Despite the critical rigor he brought to the usage of others, Freud's own text was not, however, itself free of figurative language. When, for instance, he sought to improve upon Meynert's notion of how the periphery of the body was represented in the cortex, he proposed that the sensory cortical tracts

> contain the body periphery in the same way as—to borrow an example from the subject with which we are concerned here—a poem contains the alphabet, i.e., in a completely different arrangement serving other purposes, in manifold associations of the individual elements, whereby some may be represented several times, others not at all.[30]

This was a "mere" metaphor: a deliberate use of figurative language to elucidate an obscure point. But elsewhere in Freud's text metaphor was present in subtler, but also more pervasive and influential forms. At one point Freud declared: "The whole organization of the brain seems to fall into two central apparatuses of which the cerebral cortex is the younger, while the older one is repesented by the ganglia of the forebrain which have still maintained some of their functions."[31] The brain is here endowed with a biography; it is made up of both "older" and "younger" parts. The allusion is, of course, to an evolutionary theory that depicted contemporary bodily organs as the product of a long process of elaboration. But this is only to say that Freud drew upon a resource already saturated with metaphors derived from an analogy with the individual life cycle.

Moreover, Freud avowed that:

> "[i]n assessing the functions of the speech apparatus under pathological conditions we are adopting as a guiding principle Hughlings Jackson's doctrine that all these modes of reaction represent instances of functional retrogression . . . of a highly organized apparatus, and therefore correspond to earlier states of its functional development.

---

[29] Compare the contrasting models present in nineteenth-century French ecological thought described by Paul Rabinow, *French Modern: Norms and Forms of the Social Environment* (Chicago: Chicago University Press, 1989), pp. 128–29.

[30] Ibid., p. 53 [55].

[31] Ibid., pp. 49–50 [51]. Translation slightly modified.

Within this economy, the newer forms of nervous arrangement and functioning were also "higher" than the older; and it was these more recent acquisitions that were most vulnerable.[32] A system of values was thus insinuated into an overtly naturalistic text. We have already seen how ideologically charged this set of figurative oppositions was (see chapter 4).

Freud did not therefore escape the prison house of language. What his text does reveal is a shift away from certain metaphorical understandings of the nervous system accompanied by the assimilation of other models. Put crudely, instead of a preoccupation with mapping function in *space* was put the endeavor to locate it in various temporal series. While for classical aphasiology the disease was to be understood as the perturbation of a timeless extended mechanism best represented by a diagram, now it was seen as explicable only in terms of the epic narrative of the unfolding of the nervous system. Dysfunction was proof that time's arrow could point in either direction.

Freud's text is also marked by the display of a new note of humility in the face of the difficulty of the subject he essays. There is almost a sense of awe at the complexity and subtlety of the cerebral mechanisms underlying the functions of language. This sense of the immense—perhaps insurmountable—obstacles facing anyone seeking to give an account of these operations is in contrast to the confidence of an earlier generation of investigator. The implication is that all proposed answers to these questions must be to some degree unsatisfactory and always provisional; the goal of a final and comprehensive map of the brain was spurious.

Marie's *Travaux et Mémoires*

When contemporaries sought a single iconic figure for the reaction against classical aphasiology that took place at the turn of the twentieth century they usually settled on Pierre Marie. This personality was endowed with dramatic, almost heroic attributes: he was the iconoclast, a destroyer of worlds and a shaker of complacency; but he was also the architect of a new strikingly original edifice. To a remarkable degree, therefore, Marie's doctrines and influence on the field were intertwined with and seen to derive from his character. There is an obvious analogy with Henry Head's depiction of that other revolutionary, John Hughlings Jackson—as well as with Head's self-fashioning.

[32] On Freud's borrowings from Jackson see: Frank J. Sulloway, *Freud, Biologist of the Mind: Beyond the Psychoanalytic Legend* (Bungay: Fontana, 1980), pp. 270–272; S. P. Fullinwider, "Sigmund Freud, John Hughlings Jackson, and Speech," *Journal of the History of Ideas* 44 (1983): 151–158.

This image was largely derived from a series of three articles published between May and November 1906 in the *Semaine Médicale*; these along with a number of other writings on aphasia were in 1926 republished as volume 1 of Marie's *Travaux et Mémoires*. They are highly polemical texts designed to discredit by means of a variety of rhetorical devices the works of others while proposing a fresh understanding of aphasia. But what is equally striking is the way in which these documents also project a depiction of their author; even at source, therefore, the man and the ideas are inseparable. The title can be read as adverting "labours and memories" of an individual as well as to a body of works and memoirs.

This characteristic is among the most distinctive aspects of Marie's writing; it is also one sign of his deviance. A properly composed contribution to scientific discourse was supposed to be distinguished by an *effacement* of the self (see chapter 1). Quite apart from their conceptual content Marie's text thus challenged some of the defining conventions of classical aphasia studies. Instead of purveying observations and theories as if they were the effects of a generalized gaze and disembodied consciousness, Marie's status as a concrete historical actor with a perspective conditioned by his biography was inscribed into his text. "I have had," he declared,

> the very great honour of being Broca's and Charcot's intern; I have therefore been brought up to believe in cerebral localizations. At the moment when I arrived at the Salpêtrière, my master Charcot delivered his famous lectures on aphasia; it was to me (and even now I am very proud of this choice) that he confided the responsibility of presenting a kind of critical compendium of his opinions; indeed, it was I who, on this occasion, composed a diagram of the various language centres that has become almost classic.[33]

Marie thus established a definite and significant place for himself in the history of aphasia studies. His pedagogic background made it all the more remarkable that Marie was now the most ardent critic of the doctrines of his former masters; there was, indeed, a piquant irony in the fact that he was engaged in deconstructing an edifice to which he had as a student made a modest but enduring contribution. The conspicuous result of that contribution was one of aphasiology's most famous diagrams.

The reasons for this volte-face were also to be found in the details of Marie's biography. When in 1895 he took up the post at the infirmary of the Bicêtre he was presented with the opportunity to pursue his own in-

---

[33] Pierre Marie, *Travaux et mémoires*, 2 vols. (Paris: Masson, 1926), vol. 1, p. 94. On Marie's involvement with the Charcot school see: Christopher G. Goetz, Michel Bonduelle, Toby Gelfand, *Charcot: Constructing Neurology* (New York: Oxford University Press, 1995), especially pp. 320–21.

tensive investigations into the subject of aphasia. At first, he remained a "loyal disciple":

> I strove to classify the cases I encountered in one or the other of the classic categories, but as my methods of clinical investigation became more minute and more exact, I found to my great astonishment and also to my great displeasure that the patients I observed did not conform to authors' descriptions, or at least did so only in a very imperfect fashion. The clinical picture of aphasia appears very different depending on whether one studies it in books or in nature.[34]

Marie thus suffered a crisis of faith in the creed in which he had been educated.

This anecdote sketches some of the most salient characteristics of the authorial self that inhabits Marie's text. In the first place, this is an independent *moi* distinguished by his autonomy of judgment: not even early indoctrination could prevent Marie from eventually forming his own opinions. Second, in this and in other instances he insists upon his preference for personal experience as a source of truth. In particular, observations must always take precedence over mere reasoning; he complained that some of his colleagues had proceeded as if "the logic of men did not lag far behind the logic of things and could take the place of direct observation."[35]

Third, this ostentatious empiricism leads to an antipathy for system and dogma. The "book" serves as a metonym for all received authority that distracts the mind from its lonely search for truth. "If we wish to acquire true notions of aphasia," Marie declared, "it is necessary to disregard all we have read and learned about word images, about aphasias of reception and conduction, about language centres, etc., etc.; we must confine ourselves to examining the facts without preconception."[36] Above all, the inquiring mind needed to disencumber itself of the trammels imposed on its independent judgment by the "classic doctrines" embodied in the writings of "classic authors."[37]

The self inserted into the text is, in short, jealous of its autonomy, hostile to authority, suspicious of system, and inclined to prefer fact to mere reason. It is hostile to the written word as embodying an inauthentic, or at best incomplete, form of knowledge. This persona conforms closely to the type of the good scientist as portrayed by numerous nineteenth-century

---

[34] Ibid.
[35] Ibid, p. 5.
[36] Ibid.
[37] Ibid., pp. 6, 35.

expositions of the qualities required of those who aspired to penetrate the mysteries of nature. But such visions of the inquisitive, disabused, and irreverent intellect had older sources in the general literary culture. It comes as no surprise when Marie asserts that:

> Montaigne's well-known motto *"what do I know?"* should be practised by each person with respect to himself; but, when it is a matter of *DOGMAS*, of whatever nature, established or transmitted by those who went before us, is it not right to apply to these men, as fallible as we are and even more ignorant, the same motto, and to ask ourselves: *"What did they know?"* [38]

By citing Montaigne he aligned himself with a skeptical, antirationalist rendering of the self that long antedated the ideals of natural science.

Some of the other traits on display in Marie's writing are indeed either irrelevant to or even (on the conventional view) inimical to the identity of the scientist. There was, for instance, the unexpected ingredient of humor. Thus there is a lengthy anecdote about how an aphasic cook (a *good* cook) committed various comic solecisms when Marie asked him to fry an egg. The story makes a serious point: it demonstrated, according to Marie, that aphasia was not simply an affection of the language faculty; intelligence as a whole was impaired. But the narrative is constructed so as to underline the ludicrous aspects of the event.[39]

Irony is also employed liberally to make opposing doctrines appear foolish. Commenting on Jean-Baptiste Bouillaud's surmise that the faculty of language resided in the frontal half of the brain, Marie sniffed that he might well have made the right guess—"the risk was slight: only 1 in 2, as in 'rouge ou noir', 'pair ou impair'; fortune did not favour him."[40] This passage provides a good example of Marie's epigrammatic style.

The authorial self is also something of a snob. When seeking to show the degree to which aphasics remained "normal" in their behaviour, Marie remarked with approval, and perhaps relief, that "observance of social distances is an aspect of their mental life that leaves little to be desired."[41] A number of anecdotes from Marie's personal experience follow to illustrate the point. Moreover, Marie's references to the particular segment of society with which he is most intimately concerned—the medical profession—also betrays a haughty awareness of distinctions in rank and in imputed worth.

There are several references in the text to the "rabble" [*foule*] that comprises the majority of the medical corps; this mass is contrasted to a more

[38] Ibid., p. 30.
[39] Ibid., pp. 8–9.
[40] Ibid., p. 81.
[41] Ibid., p. 10.

discriminating elite. The distance between the two is not primarily one of income, but of unequal intellectual endowment. Marie suggested that the medical mob exerted an influence far in excess of its intelligence, sometimes with deleterious effects on the progress of science. Thus, speaking of the rapid success enjoyed by Broca's claims, Marie sourly observes: "the new doctrine was rapidly adopted by the medical masses while the aristocracy of the profession maintained a posture of incredulity, defiance or even hostility towards it."[42] The author's vision of the dynamics of the medical profession is a microcosm of early twentieth-century antidemocratic polemic. It reflects contemporary preoccupation with the dangers posed by the crowd.[43]

Marie is, however, a radical conservative. He is determined to tear down the proud theoretical edifice that positivist science had raised around aphasia since the 1860s by showing how rickety were the foundations of this massive structure. Chief among the devices turned to this aim is narrative: the text undermined received truths by telling stories. Above all, it subverts these dogmas by telling stories about their *origins*.

Aphasiology had, of course, its own history which had been carefully elaborated (not without controversy) since the early 1860s (see Introduction). But this was essentially a narrative of *discovery* that recounted how at a particular moment in time auspicious circumstances had made possible the recognition of certain natural truths about the relation of language to the brain. Marie now propounded a counternarrative of *artifice*. He undertook, in particular, to show the extent to which Broca's "discovery" was a matter of historical contingency; thereby he hoped to deprive these doctrines of their status as doxa, as irrefragable facts of nature. These much-touted truths were, in fact, no more than relics of particular instances of human vanity and folly. Marie's remembering of these circumstances was therefore an unwelcome cure for "genesis amnesia."[44]

Marie's principal contention was simple: Broca's interpretation of the two initial cases upon which his doctrine of the specificity of the seat of language rested was mistaken. He proposed to explain this error by placing Broca in his historical context and showing the play of influences that led him to these false conclusions. The exposition of this biographical infor-

---

[42] Ibid., p. 84.

[43] The right-wing polemicist Gustave Le Bon was, for instance, much preoccupied with the social consequences of the balance of power between the "mob" and the "elite." See: *La Psychologie politique et la défense sociale* (Paris: Ernest Flammarion, 1910), book III, chapter 1. For a discussion of this literature see: Susanna Barrows, *Distorting Mirrors: Visions of the Crowd in Late Nineteenth-Century France* (New Haven: Yale University Press, 1981); Robert A. Nye, *The Origins of Crowd Psychology: Gustave Le Bon and the Crisis of Mass Democracy in the Third Republic* (Beverly Hills: Sage, 1975).

[44] Terdimann, *Discourse*, p. 64.

mation served also to humanize the by now iconic figure of Broca and so to draw attention to the idol's feet of clay.

The first narrative thread concerned Broca's own biography. He had misinterpreted the nature of the lesion in Lelong's case because "*he did not understand the senile brain.*" Broca had been surgeon to the Bicêtre for a mere eleven months when he conducted this autopsy. By way of contrast, Marie remarked that *he* had required four years of experience "to orientate myself a little in the pathological anatomy of the senile brain—even though the autopsies of the medical service at the Bicêtre are incomparably more numerous than those of the surgical service."[45] Again Marie's personal history served to cast light on the issues in question; his presence in the text served as a touchstone.

Broca's inexperience might account for, and perhaps excuse, his error. But it did not explain how and why one man's fault had acquired the status of orthodoxy. This was a question that could not be answered merely by reference to any individual biography; it required an account of the condition of the medical community at the time and even an awareness of the wider society within which scientific debate occurred.

According to Marie the first point that had to be grasped was that in 1861 Broca was still a junior figure within the Parisian medical establishment. He was overshadowed by the far more senior and imposing Bouillaud. The latter had since the 1820s been obsessed by an *idée fixe*: his insistence that the faculty of language was to be localized in the frontal lobes of the brain. The genealogy of this notion, however, extended beyond Bouillaud himself; its true author was Franz Josef Gall.

This ascription of paternity was of strategic significance. It was easy to mock the quaint and, by the standards of Marie's audience, bizarre forms of evidence upon which Gall had relied when situating the faculty of language in the anterior part of the brain. "When one reads such rubbish," Marie snorted, "one thinks one is dreaming! And yet Gall is the direct ancestor from whom the localization of language in the third frontal [convolution] proceeds!"[46] Its dubious parenthood thus undermined the legitimacy of the doctrine.

Although comprehensively discredited by the scientific authorities of the time, Gall's system had for a quarter of a century continued to enjoy a certain vogue. Among these phrenological enthusiasts none, however, was more "dithyrambic" than Bouillaud. Not only did he himself espouse these ideas, he sought to impose them on others. Having thus set the scene—casting Bouillaud in the unmistakeable role of villain—Marie now cues Broca "to make his entrance."[47]

[45] Marie, *Travaux*, p. 72.
[46] Ibid., p. 79.
[47] Ibid., p. 81.

Marie's characterization of Broca is a good deal more complex than that allowed to Gall the buffoon or to Bouillaud the knave. When describing the debates in the *Société d'Anthropologie* Marie emphasises the judicious nature of Broca's contributions: "one cannot too much admire his discourse where his superiority to most of his contemporaries shone."[48] In other words, Broca was decidedly not of the *foule*. He was, however, lured from the path of sound reasoning by Bouillaud's auxiliary, Simon Alexandre Ernest Auburtin, who had reminded him of his father-in-law's doctrine respecting the frontal lobes. Auburtin had, moreover, challenged his auditors to find a single case of speech loss in which the frontal lobes were not affected. It was with these suggestions in mind that Broca had approached his first case of aphasia, that of Leborgne or "Tan." After the patient's death an extensive lesion of the surface of the brain was discovered; but because of the suggestions that had been fed to him, Broca chose to emphasize only the damage done to the third frontal convolution thus apparently confirming Bouillaud's thesis.[49]

Marie felt competent and confident enough to assert that, left to himself, Broca would have avoided this error because he possessed "too scientific and too precise a spirit" not to notice the other lesions.[50] He here took on the stance of an omniscient narrator whose knowledge and insight far exceeded that of the historical actors and yet who was able to excuse the errors into which they fell as the result of their peculiar historical situation.

While Broca's unfortunate suggestibility might account for his mistake, it was not a sufficient explanation for the success that his new doctrine subsequently enjoyed in the medical community. It was at this juncture that the malign influence of *la foule* made itself felt. Bouillaud was able to mobilize a crowd of students and partisans of phrenology in support of the alleged localization. These were the "medical masses" who enthusiastically embraced the innovation while the elite of the profession showed its superior wisdom by remaining skeptical. There is no attempt to conceal the author's aristocratic contempt for the "army" recruited to this cause:

> It was the *mob*, the mob with its divinatory instinct and its profound ignorance, the at once incredulous and gullible mob, especially if in the object of their belief there is something of the extraordinary and the marvelous.[51]

---

[48] Ibid., p. 82.

[49] Ibid., pp. 82–83.

[50] Ibid., p. 89.

[51] Ibid., p. 90. The "army" of medical *sans culottes* Marie to whom ascribes the success of the localizationist cause may be contrasted with the "army" of scientific *facts* which Bouillaud himself claimed to have mustered: see p. 92. It is the debased humanity of the former army that discredits the victory the doctrine achieved.

It was, moreover, possible to analyze further the psychology and motivation of this localizationist rabble when due attention was paid to the cultural context in which the new doctrine had been received. At that time there was, Marie pointed out, a

> fierce struggle between spiritualism on the one hand and materialism on the other, for it was under that name that some sought to stigmatize free thought. Now for the pure spiritualists it seemed that there was something derogatory to the dignity of the human spirit in the doctrine that purported to circumscribe in certain fixed points of the brain this or that mental faculty.—One can also easily imagine how keenly all the progressives [*novateurs*] defended the localizationist theory which, were they to triumph, should, in their opinion, undermine the foundations of the old philosophy.

Moreover, "political passions were also involved, and, among the students, faith in localizations was virtually part of the republican credo."[52]

There is an awareness here of the political import of the localization debates of the 1860s. In particular, the role of the new ideas of the distribution of function in the brain in the republican way of thinking is clearly registered (see chapter 2). What is, however, most striking about the passage is the posture of detachment that Marie adopts towards these conflicts between competing worldviews. His vantage point as an historian allows him to identify the ideological influences upon these scientific debates better than the participants themselves; but he feels no need to take sides. He is *superior* to these struggles and able to appreciate the ironies of the clash of armies that were only dimly aware of the nature of the cause for which they contended.

Marie's text thus uses narrative to destabilize the "dogma" he sought to discredit. His was not so much an historical sociology of knowledge as of error. By finding sufficient causes for their actions and conclusions in the biographies and historical circumstances of the individuals concerned in formulating and promulgating the localizationist doctrine, Marie deprived these beliefs of the spurious status of irrefragable truth. They were merely *beliefs* contingent on the historical perspectives of those who held them. The author's ability to perceive this play of forces upon the actions of Broca and his contemporaries was itself a token of his transcendence of such historical contingency; Marie was free of all such extraneous influences and able to perceive a pristine nature and to judge doctrines without distortion or prejudice. *His* judgment was untainted by personal or social interest.

To underline his immunity to the all too human weaknesses and partialities of others, as well as the independence of his judgment, Marie's favored

---

[52] Ibid., p. 90.

witness to truth was not the authority of men but the mute testimony of things. In a masterly gesture rich with irony he turned the very objects upon which the localizationist edifice rested into reproaches to that dogma.

The brains of the two patients upon which Broca had based his initial claims about the localization of the faculty of language had in 1861 been deposited in the Musée Dupuytren; there they remained as trophies to the remorseless encroachment of science on the domain of the spiritual. "Their conservation," Marie declared, "leaves nothing to be desired, anyone can view them in their total integrity . . . ": no attempts had been made to section these organs.[53] The material integrity of these brains was a warrant for their integrity as witnesses; no human hand had sought to fashion them toward some partiality. The reverence with which they were treated was also an indication of their status as major scientific relics.

Marie first gave a purportedly purely descriptive account of the state of the brain of Leborgne, the first of Broca's two cases. He noted that the lesion had destroyed not only the third frontal convolution but also much of the left hemisphere including part of the zone of Wernicke (T1) and the supramarginal gyrus. Why, therefore, Marie demanded, had Broca disregarded the damage to all these other areas of the cortex and concentrated attention solely on the destruction of F3? Broca's "error" was again explicable by reference to history—in this instance the history of his discipline: at the time when he wrote certain "false ideas" were current in the field of neuropathology. Broca was simply "subservient to the ideas of his time";[54] he had failed to attain the autonomy of judgment demanded of the scientist.

Marie was in thrall to no such external authority. He merely reported the evidence of his senses which was plainly at odds with the interpretations placed upon the brains of these aphasics by Broca and his followers. To communicate conviction it was, however, necessary to allow his readers access to the same evidence before the facts he observed became self-evident to *them*. For this purpose words needed to be supplemented by pictorial forms of representation.

Marie's text offered two depictions of the brain of Leborgne. The first (fig. 6.2) was presented as an unalloyed, naturalistic rendering of the thing as it was. The rubric to the illustration took great pains to establish its credentials as a veridical image. The drawing had been made from "the photograph of the piece actually conserved at the Museum Dupuytren." There were also instructions on how this design was to be read: "One sees that, in addition to the lesion of the third frontal [convolution], the

[53] Ibid., pp. 65–66.
[54] Ibid., p. 68.

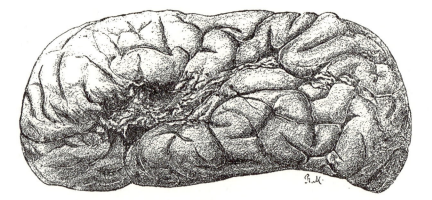

Figure 6.2. Left hemisphere of Leborgne. Pierre Marie,
Travaux et mémoires (1926)

softening exists along the entire length of the fissure of Sylvius and in consequence also extends to the zone of Wernicke."[55] As far as was possible this representation, along with its accompanying text, was to induce in the reader the effect of having immediate sight of the specimen—albeit with Marie guiding the eye.

The second representation took the form of one of the stereotyped brain profiles that had formed part of the standard repertoire of aphasia studies since the 1860s (see chapter 3). Upon this was mapped the true extent of the lesion evident in Leborgne's brain (Fig. 6.3). The rubric stressed the derivative nature of this image; it was to be compared "with the depiction of the piece itself, fig. 1." Nonetheless, this secondary figure was the more crucial to the strategic aims of the text because it demonstrated the arbitrary limitation that Broca had placed upon the localization of the lesion in his reading of the postmortem appearance. It revealed, moreover, the involvement of what Marie claimed was the true language region of the cortex. All such disputes over localization presupposed, however, an agreed topography of the cortex upon which lesions could be mapped; this Marie did not question.

Other diagrams were deployed in an equally partisan way—to show, for instance, that a case of true "Broca's aphasia" could occur without the involvement of the third frontal convolution. Conversely, this convolution could be affected without the occurrence of aphasic symptoms. The putative explanation of the occasional and accidental involvement of F3 in some cases of aphasia lay in the nature of the blood supply to various parts of the cortex. "I have," Marie explained,

[55] Ibid., p. 66.

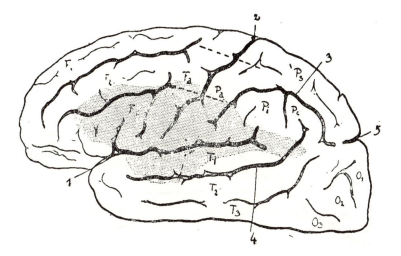

Figure 6.3. Left hemisphere of Leborgne rendered as standard brain profile.
Pierre Marie, *Travaux et mémoires* (1926)

reproduced here, so that the argument should be more easy to follow, a diagram produced by my intern François Moutier, of one of the brains from the
Laboratory, showing the distribution of the branches of the *sylvian artery* in
this brain.—One sees from this figure . . . that the artery of the third frontal
convolution is the first branch, which, on the external face of the hemisphere,
arises from the sylvian, then come the branches for the first and second temporal [convolutions].[56](fig. 6.4)

The rubric to the diagram demonstrated how, if the blood supply was
interrupted at a particular point, both T1 and F3 would be affected. Broca's aphasia would ensue; the damage done to "Broca's region" would,
however, be strictly incidental to the lesion of the temporal lobe. It was in
this part of the brain that, Marie insisted, the true cortical language center
was located. Injury here, and here alone, could produce aphasia proper.

Marie maintained that true aphasia invariably involved some loss of
comprehension of language: it was, to use the old terminology, *always*
"sensory" aphasia. What truly distinguished Broca's aphasia from the condition identified by Wernicke was that in the former an additional set of
symptoms supervened. As well as an impairment in the understanding of
language, the patient found it difficult to articulate words; Marie called
this condition *anarthria*. It was typical of Marie's style that his position
was summarized by an epigram: "Broca's aphasia = Wernicke's aphasia +

[56] Ibid., p. 108.

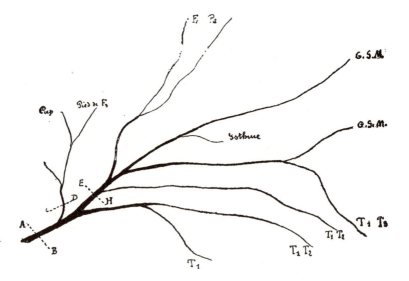

Figure 6.4. "Schematic representation, following nature, of the distribution of the branches of the sylvian artery." Pierre Marie, *Travaux et mémoires* (1926)

Anarthria."[57] It was, moreover, possible to designate the lesions responsible for this syndrome. In effect, Marie carved out a new territory in the brain to which he gave the name of the "quadrilateral" or the "lenticular zone" (fig. 6.5). Marie's claim as a namer and a discoverer was well marked in the text.[58]

The diagrams employed to make these points were varied in style and perspective. On the whole, however, Marie favored more naturalistic over schematic styles of representation. He displayed a pronounced skepticism about the heuristic worth of the numerous diagrams that were so characteristic of the text of classical aphasiology. Joseph Grasset, author of a work on *Les Centres Nerveux*, provided a convenient representative of this tendency. Marie gently mocked the "polygons" with which Grasset had sought to capture the complexities of the operations of the nervous apparatus (fig. 6.6).[59]

He conceded that such schemata might have some use in pedagogy. But they betrayed a proclivity for excessive abstraction and yearning for system that needed to be held strictly in check. The limited "masuetude" Marie was willing to allow diagrams was conceded only on certain conditions: it

---

[57] Ibid., p. 112.

[58] Ibid., pp. 111–112.

[59] Joseph Grasset, *Les centres nerveux: Physiopathologie clinique* (Paris: J.-B. Baillière, 1905), pp. 305–307.

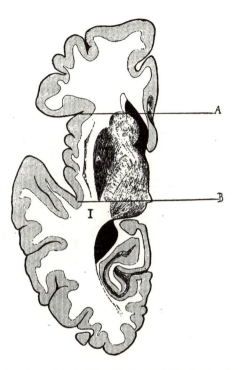

Figure 6.5. Section of the left hemisphere of the brain showing site of Marie's "lenticular zone." Pierre Marie, *Travaux et mémoires* (1926)

was wrong "to demand of diagrams more than what they could provide; "they should instead be confined exclusively to the representation of *anatomical facts* or notions derived directly from anatomical facts." On the other hand,

> to pretend to translate psychology into schemata of an anatomical kind when we know nothing, one has to admit, about the physiology and even the minute anatomy of the brain, that cannot be allowed![60]

Marie thus concluded with a skeptical and somewhat pessimistic assessment of the current state of scientific knowledge about the brain and its workings; in this respect his text approximated to the mood of Freud's. This condition of near complete ignorance would, no doubt, be ameliorated over time. But this improvement would be by way of the slow incremental accumulation of small pieces of empirical knowledge, not by bold intuitive leaps or by premature essays at systematization. Marie thus approximated to a Burkean view of progress.

[60] Marie, *Travaux*, p. 113.

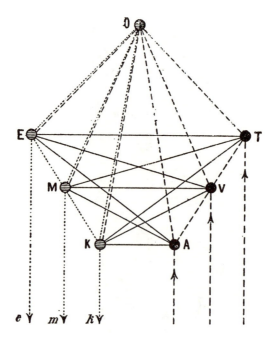

Figure 6.6. "General schema of the higher automatic centres."
Joseph Grasset, *Anatomie clinique des centres nerveux* (1902)

When in 1922 Marie reviewed the history of aphasia studies since Wernicke he once more adopted a posture of olympian condescension toward the jejune efforts of his predecessors in the field: "One could in truth call this epoch in the history of aphasia the *geometric phase*, for one does not have to look far to find neurologists working, far less with regard to the patients themselves, than with an eye to diagrams of their own invention."[61] The approximation to mathematical models of representation which had seemed the supreme achievement of classical aphasiology was thus dismissed as the most of egregious symptom of a pervasive delusion and hubris.

Bergson's *Matter and Memory*

The third dissenting text to be considered does not belong to the technical literature of neurology. It is a philosophical treatise that addresses some of the traditional issues of Western metaphysics. In his writings Henri

[61] Ibid., p. 119.

Bergson (1859–1941) challenged the dominance of nineteenth-century positivism. He proposed to supersede it with a system of thought that gave due attention to process and to lived experience. One of Bergson's chief works, *Matter and Memory* (1896), nonetheless contains a discussion of the seemingly specialist medical topic of how the clinical phenomena of aphasia are to be understood. In particular, Bergson took exception to some of the central tenets of classical aphasiology and suggested alternative ways of understanding these disorders of language. Given the intimacy— sometimes the *identity*—of language and thought in the Western tradition, this overlap between clinical and philosophical discourse is perhaps not surprising. But what gave Bergson's concern with aphasia its particular urgency was the strategic role the discourse about language and the brain had played during the second half of the nineteenth century in the generation of positivistic and naturalistic models of mind.

The debate in the Société d'Anthropologie in 1861 and the controversies that followed it were, as Pierre Marie clearly saw, the occasion for a confrontation between two worldviews that had vied for supremacy in France throughout the nineteenth century. At issue between them was the question of whether the distinction between spirit and matter, mind and body, was inviolable or whether the former categories could be collapsed into the latter. Broca's localization of the faculty of language in the brain was relevant to this conflict because it seemed to demonstrate that the noblest, definitive aspect of the human spirit had its basis in brute matter. The methodological equivalent of such claims was that there were no limits upon the explanatory scope of the natural sciences; all phenomena, including those of consciousness, were in principle capable of scientific explanation.

Bergson's *Matter and Memory* needs to be read as a response to such aggressive assertions of the primacy and sufficiency of a "physiological" understanding of the human mind.[62] In particular, Bergson's writing has to be placed in its tense relation with the works of Théodule Ribot, the most prominent spokesman of positivist psychology in nineteenth-century France.[63] In this polemic the faculty of *memory* came to occupy a

---

[62] For the context of Bergson's work see: R. C. Grogin, *The Bergsonian Controversy in France 1900–1914* (Calgary: University of Calgary Press, 1988); Sanford Schwartz, "Bergson and the Politics of Vitalism," in Frederick Burwick and Paul Douglass, *The Crisis in Modernism: Bergson and the Vitalist Controversy* (Cambridge: Cambridge University Press, 1992), pp. 277–305; Jan Goldstein, "The Advent of Psychological Modernism in France: An Alternative Narrative," in Ross, *Modernist Impulses*, pp. 190–209.

[63] For an account of Ribot's career see: John I. Brooks III, *The Eclectic Legacy: Academic Philosophy and the Human Sciences in Nineteenth-Century France* (Newark: University of Delaware Press, 1998), chapter 2. See also: Michael S. Roth, "Remembering Forgetting: *Maladies de la Mémoire* in Nineteenth-Century France," *Representations* 26 (1989): 49–68.

crucial position: above all, the way in which the elements of language were retained and recovered became a critical focus of contention.

For Ribot, "memory is, in essence, a biological fact; by accident, a psychological fact." In other words, consciousness was a late addition to a faculty of organic matter that had developed through time. The basic ability to retain and to retrieve previous impressions was an inherent property of living beings: "the bases of memory should be sought in the properties of organized matter."[64] Consciousness, according to Ribot, was a "superadded element to memory."[65]

Locating the roots of memory in organic life implied that this faculty conformed, like any other physiological function, to determinate laws.[66] These laws were most evident when the mechanisms according to which memory was regulated broke down in cases of injury or disease of the brain. Such phenomena revealed that "recollection is not . . . 'in the soul': it is fixed in its nidus, in a part of the nervous system."[67] More particularly, memories were stored in the cells of the cerebral cortex from which depository they could be retrieved when required. Ribot cited Meynert's estimate of 600,000,000 as the number of cells contained in the cortex. Given this abundance there was nothing a priori impossible about the notion that for each memory there was a dedicated cell. Memory was not therefore a unified faculty or property; it was a concatenation of individual memory traces distributed over the cerebral cortex.

The figure of the cell as a store was of course utterly commonplace—a dead metaphor, which Freud revivified in order to undermine. But Ribot supplemented this device with a more original way of conceiving how memories might be localized in the cerebral cortex:

> One can compare the modified cell to a letter of the alphabet; this letter, even while remaining the same, has combined to form the millions of words in living and dead languages. By aggregation, the most numerous and complex combinations can arise from a small number of elements.[68]

This analogy was particularly apt because this discrete embodiment was most apparent in the case of verbal memory. The "convolution of Broca" and its surrounding structures were "universally considered as the psychic

---

For an insightful account of the political valency of Ribot's psychology see: Anson Rabinbach, *The Human Motor: Energy, Fatigue, and the Origins of Modernity* (New York: Basic Books, 1990), pp. 164–167.

[64] Théodul Ribot, *Les maladies de la mémoire* (Paris: Félix Alcan, 1898), p. 4.

[65] Ibid., p. 9.

[66] Ibid., p. 2.

[67] Ibid., p. 11.

[68] Ibid., pp. 17–18.

centre for speech."[69] This localization rested upon pathological evidence; in consequence, cases of aphasia possessed in Ribot's scheme a unique exemplary value.

If his model of the particulate nature of memory was sound, then "partial amnesias" in which only part of the brain's total memory store was impaired should occur. Ribot maintained that the clinical record revealed just such selective forms of memory loss; but, "Strictly speaking, there exists only one form of partial amnesia that can be thoroughly studied: that of signs."[70]

In the avowedly "scientific" psychology that developed in the late nineteenth century, the localization and disorders of language thus occupied a privileged position. Bergson's philosophy was part of the fin de siècle reaction against the overweening pretensions of such positivist schemes. Bergson was hostile to the naturalism inherent in this project; he sought to retain a special status for mind in the material universe. He opposed mechanistic psychologies and the determinism they implied. And, in particular, he resisted the assumption that mental operations were dependent upon the material structures and physiological operations of the brain. The notion of a *spatial* representation of mind was especially inimical to Bergson's emphasis upon the centrality of time in the evolution of human consciousness.[71]

Bergson maintained that most psychologists operated with a grossly exaggerated notion of the importance of the brain. According to him, "The brain is part of the material world; the material world is not part of the brain."[72] It was absurd to imagine that perception simply "mirrored" the state of certain portions of the nervous system.

In order to diminish the brain and deprive it of the incredible properties that had been ascribed to it, Bergson emphasized the affinities between the structure and function of the nervous system and that of the "lower" elements of the nervous organization. If the brain were compared to the spinal cord, "we are bound to infer that there is merely a difference of complication, and not a difference in kind, between the functions of the brain and the reflex activity of the medullary system." Some impulses were

[69] Ibid., p. 31.

[70] Ibid., p. 113. Ribot made it clear that he was not concerned with aphasia in general, but only with that aspect of the disorder involving a partial memory loss (pp. 119–120).

[71] See: Stephen Kern, *The Culture of Time and Space 1880–1918* (Cambridge, Mass.: Harvard University Press, 1983), pp. 45–46. Henri Lefebvre has placed Bergson's writings in a nineteenth- and twentieth-century tradition of attacks upon the "primacy of the spatial." *The Production of Space*, trans. Donald Nicholson-Smith (Oxford: Blackwell, 1992), pp. 21–22.

[72] Henri Bergson, *Matter and Memory*, trans. Nancy Margaret Paul and W. Scott Palmer (London: Swan Sonnenschein, 1911 [1896]), p. 4.

mediated directly by the reflex mechanisms of the cord; others were first diverted to the brain before returning to the same spinal apparatus. Bergson demanded:

> what has it gained by this round-about course, and what did it seek in the so-called sensory cells of the cerebral cortex? I do not understand, I shall never understand, that it draws thence a miraculous power of changing itself into a representation of things; and moreover, I hold this hypothesis to be useless. . . . But what I do see clearly is that the cells of the cortex that are termed sensory . . . allow the stimulation received to reach *at will* this or that motor mechanism of the spinal cord, and so to *choose* its effect.[73]

The addition of a cortical component to the nervous process therefore allowed for more complex and selective movements; it did not constitute a basis for consciousness. It was an error to imagine "the nervous system as a separate being, of which the function is, first, to elaborate perceptions, and then to create movements. The truth is that my nervous system, interposed between the objects which affect my body and those which I can influence, is a mere conductor, transmitting, sending back, or inhibiting movement."[74]

This assertion had obvious consequences for understanding the nature and modalities of memory. If it were true that "the necessary and sufficient cause of perception lies in a certain activity of the brain, this same cerebral activity, repeating itself more or less completely in the absence of the object, will suffice to reproduce perception; memory will be entirely explicable by the brain."[75] But, in truth, all that could be laid down in the brain were schemata for the performance of certain movements; the body "can neither beget or cause an intellectual state."[76] Perceptual memory must have a different locus.

Bergson thus took upon himself the task of ascertaining where "in the operations of memory, the office of the body begins, and where it ends."[77] He ascribed to the nervous system the strictly limited task of acting as an intermediary between sensation and motion, while regarding "memory itself as absolutely independent of matter."[78] To secure this position it was necessary to show the fallacy of the physical theories of perception memory that had previously prevailed.

These mistaken theories were largely based on false metaphors for the processes in question. One difficulty

---

[73] Ibid., p. 19.
[74] Ibid., p. 40.
[75] Ibid., p. 84.
[76] Ibid., p. 233.
[77] Ibid., p. 85.
[78] Ibid., p. 232.

arises from the fact that we imagine perception to be a kind of photographic view of things, taken from a fixed point by that special apparatus which is called an organ of perception—a photograph which would then be developed in the brain-matter by some unknown chemical and psychical process of elaboration.

But, Bergson objected, if there was indeed such a photograph it already existed "in the very heart of things"; it did not need to be elaborated in the brain and there was no black screen on which it could be projected.[79]

The ruling metaphors of memory were equally flawed. Bergson was, in particular, concerned to discredit "the strange hypothesis of recollections stored in the brain, which are supposed to become conscious as though by a miracle, and bring us back to the past by a process that is left unexplained."[80] Bergson acknowledged that certain well-established facts could be adduced in support of this way of conceiving the mechanisms of memory. Above all, there were "the cerebral lesions which seem to bring about a destruction of memories; more particulary, in the case we are studying, there are lesions of the brain found in word deafness."[81] Indeed, cases of sensory aphasia provided the one and only instance which seemed to support the view that memory consisted in the form of cerebral deposits. At this juncture clinical and philosophical discourse intersected.

Bergson's strategy was similar to that of Freud, although its intent was quite different. He focussed attention upon the figurative nature of the notion of the existence within the cortex of "slumbering" auditory memories waiting for a stimulus capable of arousing them. When it was subjected to scrutiny it was easy enough to find anomalies and absurdities in this figure. One could imagine how an object might be stored at some local site. But "a word is not an object with well-defined outlines; for the same word pronounced by different voices, or by the same voice on different notes, gives a different sound." Were there then as many "word images" stored up as there were possible permutations of any given word? If so, how did the brain choose between them: "For you must bear in mind that this memory is supposed to be an inert and passive thing and consequently incapable of discovering, beneath external differences, an internal similitude."?[82]

The ruling metaphor of memory broke down precisely because of its inability to cope with the element of intelligent, purposive choice involved in recollection:

[79] Ibid., p. 31.
[80] Ibid., p. 104.
[81] Ibid., p. 146.
[82] Ibid., p. 147.

I grant that the memory of a word will be called up by the sound of that word: yet it is necessary, for this, that the sound of the word should have been heard by the ear. How can the sounds perceived speak to memory, how can they choose, in the storehouse of auditory images, those which should come to rejoin them, unless they have been already separated, distinguished,—in short, perceived,—as syllables and as words?[83]

The failure of theorists of sensory aphasia to appreciate this necessary psychic element to the apprehension of auditory stimuli had, Bergson argued, vitiated much of what had been written about that disorder.

Moreover, the clinical manifestations of aphasia themselves militated against the prevalent model of how word memories were conserved and recovered. If these memories were indeed "deposited" in the cortical cells, "we should find in sensory aphasia . . . the irreparable loss of certain determined words, the integral conservation of others." More usually, however, "it is . . . the function which is diminished and not the number of recollections."[84] Moreover, the topographic model ignored certain temporal aspects of the syndrome; for instance, the fact that certain parts of speech were consistently more vulnerable to loss than others. This could hardly be explained on the hypothesis that "verbal images were really deposited in the cells of the cortex: it would be wonderful indeed that disease should always attack these cells in the same order."[85] This crux was symptomatic of a fundamental problem of the physicalist understanding of memory: its attempt to congeal into distinct and independent particles the flux of a continuous undivided process.[86]

Bergson maintained that this weakness was manifest in the history of the diagrams characteristic of classical aphasia studies. These had sought to represent the elements of the language process as so many "stations" between which a finite number of lines of communication operated. But "each new fact will force us to complicate our diagram, to insert new stations along the line of the movement; and yet all these stations laid side by side will never be able to reconstitute the movement itself." Neurology itself, Berson noted, was becoming "more sceptical with regard to diagrams, [and] returning purely and simply to the description of facts."[87]

Bergson's conclusion was thus that it was "vain . . . to treat memory-images and ideas as ready-made things, and then assign to them an abiding place in problematical centres."[88] In fact, all that could be embodied in

[83] Ibid., p. 135.
[84] Ibid., p. 149.
[85] Ibid., pp. 151–152.
[86] Ibid., p. 156.
[87] Ibid., pp. 156, 158.
[88] Ibid., p. 159.

the brain were "motor diagrams" that enabled a memory to actualize itself as a movement. The "alleged destruction of memories by an injury to the brain is but a break in the continuous progress by which [memories] actualize themselves."[89]

But if the figure of "the brain as a storehouse of memories" was to be rejected what was to be put in its place? Bergson suggested an analogy between the auditory region of the brain and a sense organ. The latter could be compared to an "immense keyboard, on which the external object executes at once its harmony of a thousand notes" thus eliciting a sensation. Similarly, the temporal region could be considered a "mental ear" from which the same sensations could be called up in the absence of external stimulus. A keyboard, however, required a player in the form of some "purely psychical cause."[90]

Establishing the existence of this immaterial player was Bergson's principal concern. He maintained that:

> there is one, and only one, method of refuting materialism: it is to show that matter is precisely that which it appears to be. Thereby we eliminate all virtuality, all hidden power, from matter, and establish the phenomena of spirit as an independent reality.[91]

The question of memory possessed a "capital importance" because this faculty had been so entirely incorporated by those propounding a physicalist understanding of mind. It was therefore necessary to demonstrate that "memory must be, in principle, a power absolutely independent of matter. . . . And hence any attempt to derive pure memory from an operation of the brain should reveal on analysis a radical illusion."[92]

Bergson expressed ethical and aesthetic reasons for why it was so important to insist upon the separate status of memory and to resist any attempt to explain it as a function of the brain. He found repugnant the necessitarian implications of any account that tied memory (and by implication all processes of consciousness) to the workings of some cerebral mechanism. It was imperative to preserve a role for the spontaneous and creative action of spirit in the world; to maintain the mind's capacity to add "something new to the universe and to its history."[93] In places this concern is expressed in more lyrical terms: "To call up the past in the form of an image, we must be able to withdraw ourselves from the action of the

---

[89] Ibid., p. 160.
[90] Ibid., pp. 165–166.
[91] Ibid., p. 80.
[92] Ibid., pp. 80–81.
[93] Ibid., pp. 2–3.

moment, we must have the power to value the useless, we must have the will to dream."[94]

Because Ribot and his like had placed such emphasis upon the facts of neuropathology as evidence for their own mechanistic view of memory, Bergson too was obliged to address the discourse of aphasia. He subjected the ruling metaphors of the discipline to scrutiny in order to expose their arbitrary, artificial character. Bergson's own preferred metaphor for the interrelation of mind and brain was, however, more revealing than perhaps he imagined. It harked back to venerable figures of the body as an instrument of an immaterial entity that somehow constituted the human essence. The brain was, moreover, likened to a *musical* instrument; its spiritual player was engaged in a creative exercise directed toward aesthetic rather than merely practical ends. While Bergson was content for the brain to be the store for the "motor mechanisms" necessary to orientate the body in its mundane activities, he insisted on the existence of a separate category of spontaneity where, from a narrowly utilitarian point of view, entirely *useless* forms of mentation could occur. He sought a cosmos in which bourgeois values did not hold exclusive sway, where the machine was not god: a universe in which the dreamer, the artist, and the philosopher would have a place.[95]

. . . . . .

According to Henri Lefebvre,

> around 1910 a certain space was shattered. It was the space of common sense, of knowledge (*savoir*), of social practice, of political power, a space hitherto enshrined in everyday discourse, just as in abstract thought. As the environment and channel for communications; the space, too, of classical perspective and geometry, developed from the Renaissance onwards on the basis of the Greek tradition . . . and bodied forth in Western art and philosophy.[96]

It is tempting, on the basis of the texts discussed above, to conclude that among the casualties of this seismic event was the space of classical nineteenth-century aphasia studies. After the strictures of Freud, Marie, and Bergson, it was, surely, impossible ever again to imagine that the processes of language could be represented by a quasi-geometric design.

A full cultural history of early twentieth-century neurology would seek to place developments in this seemingly esoteric realm within the context

[94] Ibid., p. 94.

[95] For the cultural context of this reaction against the "materialism" (in all senses of the word) of nineteenth-century society see: Grogin, *Bergsonian Controversy*, especially chapter 1.

[96] Lefebvre, *The Production*, p. 25.

of more general cultural reorientations. It would, for instance, explore the obvious resonances between Pierre Marie's iconoclasm and the "quest for liberation, . . . break, in aesthetic and moral terms, from central authority, from patriarchy, from bourgeois conformity"[97] prevalent in the Paris of his day. Eksteins and other historians of the period have pointed to the importance of the Great War in consolidating modernist sensibility. We have seen how for Henry Head and others the war was indeed seen as a watershed in the understanding of the brain and of its workings in health and disease; their attempts to realize this conviction in the period after 1918 would be a fruitful subject for further study.

While accepting that it is possible to find evidence for a reorientation in neurological thinking around the turn of the twentieth century (Lefebvre's "around 1910" has to be interpreted generously), a note of caution is indicated. Classical aphasiology was not simply a set of texts; it was a body of practice grounded in the technologies of the clinic. Its literary apparatus was merely the end product and the most durable relic of those patterns of work. The success of the enterprise was predicated on a certain blindness to other ways of knowing; the likes of Freud and Marie achieved their effects chiefly by drawing attention to those occlusions. It would be fanciful, however, to imagine that the appearance of a few, or several, aberrant texts could dismantle or deflect the great engine that Paul Broca had set in motion.[98] Rather like innovative chess grandmasters, the neurological iconoclasts were seeking novel variations, original ways of playing a game to whose fundamentals they remained committed.

---

[97] Morris Eksteins, *Rites of Spring: The Great War and the Birth of the Modern Age* (London: Bantam Press, 1989), p. 48.

[98] To avoid any misunderstanding: it would be perhaps more apt to say that the primed engine set Broca in motion.

SEVEN

MAKING GOOD

How are we to proceed with a patient who is *speechless?*
(Kurt Goldstein, Die Behandlung, Fürsorge un
Gegutachtung der Gehirn Verletzungen, *p. 75.)*

B
Y THE EARLY DECADES of the twentieth century a vast body
of writing existed on many aspects of the subject of aphasia, notably on its symptomatology and physiopathology. This archive was
both rich and complex, encompassing ever more intricate aspects of the
subject. A number of authors came to remark, however, on a remarkable
lacuna within this wealth of texts. In 1914, for instance, Hugo Stern
pointed out that large as the literature on aphasia was, "the actual therapeutic side of the question is relatively little discussed and comparatively
scant attention is paid to the interests of the patient."[1]

Stern acknowledged that this generalization needed to be qualified.
Some of the classic authors in the field *had* given some attention to the
question of therapy. Indeed, this was true of Paul Broca himself, whose
writings were fundamental to the literature on aphasia. In 1865 Broca
described his attempts to treat a patient who could neither speak nor write
by presenting him with an alphabet and trying to teach him to recognize
letters. Subsequently Broca attempted to get this "aphemic" to assemble
these letters into syllables and then words. He conceded that his efforts
to rehabilitate this patient met with little success.[2]

Such occasional forays into treatment did not, however, constitute a
sustained or systematic effort to develop strategies to alleviate the aphasic's
symptoms. Often, indeed, it is unclear from such accounts whether relieving the patient, as opposed to gaining additional insights into his or her
condition, was the point of the exercise.[3] For the most part, the aphasic
was more an object of contemplation than a field for intervention. In this
regard aphasia typified a partiality in the progress scientific medicine had

[1] Hugo Stern, "Die Grundprinzipien der sprachärtztlichen Behandlung Aphasischer,"
Wiener Medizinische Wochenschrift 7 (1914): 247–55, p. 247.
[2] Paul Broca, "Sur le siège de la faculté du langage articulé," *Bulletins de la Société
d'Anthropologie de Paris* 6 (1865): 377–93, pp. 391–92.
[3] See, for example, the ambivalent status of the reading exercises required of a patient
suffering from "verbal blindness" in one of Charcot's cases. Désiré Bernard, *De l'aphasie et
de ses diverses formes*, 2nd ed. (Paris: Lecrosnier et Babé, 1889), pp. 76–81.

made in the nineteenth century, which after 1900 began to seem anomalous; while theoretical and experimental advances had been impressive, in nonsurgical fields comparatively little had been done to improve methods of treatment.[4]

After 1900 the small space allotted to therapy within the aphasiological canon began to seem anomalous. The neglect of therapy was explained by reference to a widespread assumption that aphasia was an incurable condition; efforts at therapy were therefore futile. Early twentieth-century criticism of this stance tended to associate it with the "anatomical" bias of the neurologists of an earlier epoch. As long as it was assumed that aphasia was the result of permanent damage to the brain's language "centers" or to the commissures connecting them, there were scant grounds for hoping that lost functions could be restored. Dominant patterns of medical language were therefore seen to constrain action. Thus Wladimir Eliasberg in 1924 remarked that: "The history of aphasia treatment is a contribution to the psychology of the medical men who have dealt with aphasia."[5] So long as "anatomical-localizationist" interests—as typified by the work of Carl Wernicke—were dominant, therapeutic concerns were accorded little importance. The focus was upon the material substrate of language, and the basic premise of these workers was "what the focal lesion has destroyed can never be restored."[6] Latterly, however, a more "psychological" approach had arisen which was more aware of the plasticity of the mental functions and thus more willing to seek ways to restore at least some level of competence to brain-damaged patients.[7]

Such veiled or overt criticism of earlier approaches tended to underestimate the sophistication of the models developed by the "anatomical" school. Nineteenth-century neurology recognized that the centers of the brain possessed considerable capacity for spontaneous recovery provided that the damage to them was not too extensive. Moreover, even if a center were irreparably impaired by injury or disease, other mechanisms might be brought into play. In particular, because the brain possessed two cerebral hemispheres while language was normally represented only unilaterally, there was scope for recovery if this spare capacity could be called into action. In Broca's words, "it seems that if the right hemisphere remains healthy, it can always take over speech in place of the left hemisphere which has been rendered impotent by a lesion."[8]

---

[4] Fritz Mohr, *Psychophysische Behandlungsmethoden* (Leipzig: S. Hirzel, 1925), p. ix.

[5] W. Eliasberg, "Die Praxis der Aphasiebehandlung," *Klinische Wochenschrift* 3 (1924): 234–39, p. 238.

[6] Ibid.

[7] See also: Fritz Mohr, "Zur Behandlung der Aphasie," *Archiv für Psychiatrie und Nervenkrankheiten* 39 (1905): 1004–1069, p. 1006.

[8] Broca, "Sur le siège," p. 389.

It was the arch diagram maker, Henry Charlton Bastian, who most fully explored the routes by which restitution of lost language function might occur. Bastian distinguished between two possible forms of amelioration. *Restitution* of the function of a center whether spontaneously or with the assistance of some medical intervention usually occurred within a short period of the onset of the malady. On the other hand, functional *compensation* occurred over a much longer span of time, sometimes over a period of years. He defined compensation as a process whereby:

> existing centres are knitted together in previously unaccustomed ways (for new modes of functional activity) coincidently with the development of new sets of commissural fibres; or else centres hitherto of comparatively low organisation and slight activity, gradually take on a higher organisation and a greatly developed functional vigour; or, again, these two processes may occur in association.[9]

Bastian duly provided several diagrams designed to demonstrate how recovery might occur through the development of new pathways and the augmentation of the capacity and activity of previously unused cortical organs.[10]

Given this understanding of the recuperative powers of the brain, the goals of therapy were clear. Treatment should be guided by two considerations: "first, as to the best means for bringing about functional restitution; and, secondly, when all that is possible has been done, or is being done, in that direction to do all in our power that may be calculated to further functional compensation."[11] The prevalent model of brain function thus did not preclude the possibility of recovery; on the contrary it provided detailed accounts of how lesions of the brain might be circumvented to create new modes of operation. Moreover, although these processes of compensation were in some degree spontaneous, it was allowed that informed medical intervention could assist their progress.

The structure of late nineteenth-century aphasiology did not, therefore, of itself preclude an attention to therapy; on the contrary, a space was specifically created for such interventions. Discussions of treatment tended, however, to be relegated to an appendix to the main text. Eliasberg's assertion that, despite the efforts of various speech therapists in the late nineteenth century, until the outbreak of the First World War therapeutic "nihilism" reigned, was essentially correct. One consequence of the experience of war, he argued, had been to renew interest in "psychological

---

[9] H. Charlton Bastian, *Aphasia and Other Speech Defects* (London: H. K. Lewis, 1898), p. 341.

[10] Ibid., pp. 264–66, 352, 357.

[11] Ibid., p. 338.

therapy."[12] The same kind of sharp before/after dichotomy that permeated Henry Head's history of his discipline is again evident (see chapter 5).

Within the overall body of nineteenth- and early twentieth-century aphasia studies therapeutics thus occupies a small and marginal position. An examination of this literature is nonetheless rewarding precisely because of its anomalous status within the canon. These texts reveal representations of the aphasic and of the medical men who encountered him that are absent elsewhere. In contrast to the bleakness and resignation characteristic of most of the literature, moreover, these works offer narratives of hope and achievement. There were, however, different ways of assaying the treatment of aphasia; in each of these patient and doctor appeared in a variety of guises.

Heroic Measures

Discussions of aphasia therapy tended to distinguish between the general and the more specific aspects of the undertaking. Care had to be paid to the general health of the patient in order to bolster his or her recuperative powers; measures should also be taken to remove the underlying causes of the symptoms. These efforts might be medical in nature. If, for instance, aphasia was the result of a thrombosis, "The physician will direct his efforts toward lessening the coagulability of the blood and preventing the extension of the thrombotic process. For this purpose the alkaline citrate or citric acid may be exhibited with advantage." When inflammation lay at the root of the problem, a more general regimen was indicated:

> Where the disease is febrile in character, rest in bed, continued for a week or more after the cessation of the fever, is essential. Any simple aperient should be used regularly. A liquid diet is desirable, and small doses of the tincture of aconite, or of salicin or salol, may be administered. Urotropin may be given empirically. It is questionable whether counterirritation over the nape of the neck or behind the ears is of any efficacy. Sometimes repeated lumbar puncture may be of value. Once the acute stage is over treatment must be pursued on general lines, and as the patient is often rather prostrated, due regard must be had to the matter of stimulation.[13]

In certain cases, however, there were severe limits to what the physician could do. In particular, "The medical treatment of intracranial tumors is practically valueless." Even when these tumors were gummatous in nature

[12] Eliasberg, "Die Praxis," p. 238.

[13] William A. White and Smith Ely Jellife, *The Modern Treatment of Nervous and Mental Diseases*, 2 vols. (London: Henry Kimpton, 1913), vol. 2, p. 488.

antisyphilitic specifics tended to yield little benefit. In such cases, "One must . . . look to the surgeon for assistance."[14]

Surgical intervention constituted the most direct and dramatic means of relieving the aphasic. It emerged as a practicable option during the 1880s.[15] This development was often portrayed in triumphant terms as indicative of the seemingly limitless scope for medical intervention; even the living brain, which had for so long been beyond the surgeon's reach, could now be touched and altered. There could be no more potent symbol of the present extent and scope for the future progress of medical science.

The Glasgow surgeon William Macewen (1848–1924), one of the early pioneers—according to some, the "father"—of intracranial surgery, in an address to the 1888 meeting of the British Medical Association listed the changes that had made possible this extension of medical potency. Macewen's address also served to establish his claims to paternity; a contemporary recalled that this occasion was crucial in the shaping of Macewen's public persona:

> Although his reception was not good at the commencement of his address, he held the audience as he unfolded his story, and when he finished, he had made a chapter in surgical history, and his own place in the temple of fame. By general acclamation Macewen that day stepped into the very front rank of surgeons.[16]

Macewen's historical narrative thus served to fashion an image of himself as a prime mover in the surgical conquest of the brain.[17]

In the past autopsy had often revealed cerebral lesions within easy range of the surgical knife. Surgeons had, however, been deterred in part by the dangers of sepsis attending operations on the brain. During his tenure as a surgeon at the Glasgow Royal Infirmary between 1877 and 1892 Macewen had begun to break down the inhibitions that had deterred his colleagues. While Joseph Lister's researches into antisepsis had done much

[14] Ibid.

[15] See: Samuel H. Greenblatt, "Cerebral Localization from Theory to Practice: Paul Broca and Hughlings Jackson to David Ferrier and William Macewen," in Samuel H. Greenblatt, T. Forchi Dagi and Mel H. Epstein (eds.), *A History of Neurosurgery in Its Scientific and Professional Contexts* (Park Ridge: American Association of Neurosurgeons, 1997), pp. 137–52.

[16] J. H. Pringle, "Sir William Macewen," *British Medical Journal* 1 (1924): 603–5, p. 603.

[17] Macewen recounted an anecdote to show that this image had achieved currency in the general population of Glasgow as well as among the medical profession. He reported being accosted at a railway station by a marble cutter who demanded that the "Professor should open his head." It later transpired that the man was suffering from a subdural hemorrhage. William Macewen, "President's Address on Brain Surgery," *British Medical Journal* 2 (1922): 155–65, p. 161.

to relieve anxiety about operating on other parts of the body, Macewen took credit to himself for overcoming the prejudice that the skull formed an impenetrable barrier to the surgeon:

> Experience gained by me showed, that not only compound fractures of the skull, but large osseous defects in the cranial vault, accompanied by extensive loss of cerebral substance, were quite amenable to treatment, exhibiting no tendency to inflammatory action, as long as the tissues were preserved aseptic. When this held true of the rough and often septic lesions produced by machinery accidents, how much surer would well planned and carefully executed operations be?[18]

Lister's original experiments in surgical antisepsis had been accompanied by various theoretical understandings of the role of microscopic organisms in causing sepsis and inflammation.[19] Macewen's account, however, is decidedly empiricist in tone: *experience* and, in particular, his *own* experience had been crucial in generating a confidence that surgery on the brain could be safely undertaken.[20] But he also maintained that such practical insights could not of themselves have made possible the neurosurgical project.

In the previous epoch, "the brain was a dark continent, in which [surgeons] could descry neither path or guide capable of leading them to a particular diseased area, and, did they attempt to reach it, it could only be by groping in the dark." The source of the "light" that eventually dispelled this gloom had been the growth of physiological knowledge in the latter part of the nineteenth century. Above all,

> Broca, in 1861, from observation on human pathology, isolated a particular limited area as the seat of the faculty of articulate language. This very important investigation foreshadowed the localisation of function in other cortical centres. . . . Broca's discovery was thoroughly iconoclastic, it shook the notion entertained regarding the unity of brain function to its foundation, it awakened thought, and made men explore anew with critical eyes, fields which previously investigators were supposed to have exhausted.[21]

[18] William Macewen, "The Surgery of the Brain and Spinal Cord," *British Medical Journal* 2 (1888): 302–9, p. 302.

[19] See: Christopher Lawrence and Richard Dixey, "Practising on Principle: Joseph Lister and the Germ Theory of Disease," in Christopher Lawrence (ed.), *Medical Theory, Surgical Practice: Studies in the History of Surgery* (London: Routledge, 1992), pp. 153–215.

[20] In a later address Macewen revealed that his experience of these matters dated back to the early days of his career. "As a student at the Royal Infirmary," he recalled, "I was given the means of studying lesions in the base of the third frontal convolutions producing motor aphasia. Two such cases were in the medical wards during these years, the lesion afterwards being verified by the autopsy." Macewen, "President's Address," p. 157.

[21] Macewen, "The Surgery," pp. 302–3.

The geographical metaphor that ran through the aphasiological project (see chapter 3) here had its extension. Just as the mapping of Africa by bold explorers had been a necessary preliminary to the penetration, conquest, and exploitation of that territory,[22] so the efforts of investigators into the localization of function had made it possible for practical men like Macewen to enter into full possession of that other dark continent, the human brain.

A progression was thus sketched from the general to the particular. The movement was from a theoretical knowledge of the brain to an understanding of the underlying reality of a specific case. The products of the endeavors of a community of scientific workers transcended, although they did not render redundant, personal experience. An acquaintance with what had been ascertained about the distribution of functional centers on the cortex was, Macewen maintained, "of the greatest diagnostic value."[23] To illustrate the point he described a case of his from 1876, *"in which the Symptoms of Focal Cerebral Disease led to Diagnosis of Lesion in Broca's Lobe."*

Macewen had encountered a case of cerebral abscess "while in possession of this knowledge"—that is, both his personal experience of the possibility of keeping cerebral wounds free of infection *and* "the extended physiological knowledge" now available. The combination of right side hemiplegia and the fact that the patient was aphasic convinced Macewen that the lesion was situated "in the immediate vicinity of Broca's lobe." Confident both of his diagnosis and of his ability to operate without provoking sepsis Macewen had proposed to expose that part of the brain and to evacuate the abscess. He failed, however, to gain the support of his colleagues and the patient's parents refused to assent to the procedure. Death followed shortly afterwards, and an autopsy confirmed that the lesion was where Macewen had predicted; he appended a sketch of the brain with its lesion by way of corroboration.

He recorded his memory of the moment of revelation in some detail recalling that when "an instrument was introduced through the frontal convolution for half an inch, . . . pus flowed through the incision, proving the accuracy of the diagnosis and giving poignancy to the regret that the operation had not been permitted during life."[24] The narrative thus pro-

[22] As one leading French colonialist put it: "An officer who has successfully drawn an exact ethnographic map of the territory he commands is close to achieving complete pacification, soon to be followed by the form of organization he judges most appropriate." Quoted in Paul Rabinow, *French Modern: Norms and Forms of the Social Environment* (Chicago: Chicago University Press, 1989), p. 147. In this context, Rabinow notes, "ethnography . . . [meant] little more than the geographical location of groups."

[23] Macewen, "The Surgery," p. 303.

[24] Ibid.

vided a vindication of the reliability of the "extended physiological knowledge" (and, incidentally, of Macewen's judgment) together with a muted indictment of those who failed to trust the surgeon who wielded these resources. The tragic outcome of the story arose out of a lack of faith on the part of both the patient's friends and other medical men in the power of science in general and in Macewen—qua embodiment of that knowledge—in particular.

But the transition from knowledge to understanding to intervention was not as straightforward as this anecdote might suggest. While he insisted on the dependency of practice on theory, Macewen also emphasised the problematic nature of the passage from one to the other. In many cases,

> the evidences of focal lesion are so distinct that a diagnosis is easy; in others they are so intricate that a prolonged and minute investigation is necessary to decipher them; while there are still others in which the signs are so perplexing that at best an approximation only can be arrived at.

The text that the clinician was obliged to read was infinitely more complex, obscure, and incomplete than that contemplated by the laboratory scientist:

> To lay bare a certain known convolution on a cerebral surface and observe the results of its stimulation, is an easier task than to take what appears to be a tangled skein of nervous phenomena, such as is presented by many lesions of the complex brain of man, and to relegate each to its true source and infer from a study of the whole what particular parts of the brain are affected.[25]

At the center of the knowledge/power nexus stood the surgeon. It was for him to untangle the skein of symptoms presenting in the clinic by combining the resources supplied by physiology with his own tact and skill to arrive at the correct diagnosis and formulate an appropriate therapeutic strategy. While stressing that surgical practice in cases of brain disease could not be determined by any a priori set of principles, no matter how well grounded, Macewen continued to insist, however, on the immediate relevance of the maps that had been so laboriously constructed over the decades. The heading he gave to one of his case reports epitomizes this conviction: "*Psychical Blindness the Key to a Lesion in the Angular Gyrus.*" This was an instance where the patient presented a complex tangle of symptoms with no external injury to indicate the site of the underlying cause. What solved the conundrum was the fact that letters were "unknown symbols to him, they conveyed no impression of their meaning, the memory of their signs was gone, it was a sealed book to him." This

---

[25] Ibid., p. 305.

was enough to convince Macewen that the lesion lay in the angular gyrus; he exposed that part of the brain revealing that part of the skull lay imbedded in the gyrus. As a result of this operation the patient "became greatly relieved in his mental state."[26]

Macewen also remarked on the theoretical importance of this case. Examples of "complete mind-blindness are rare, and the definite localisation in this case will assist indicating in man what function the anterior portion of the angular gyrus and the posterior portion of the supra-marginal convolution subserve."[27] The commerce between physiology and surgery was thus reciprocal.

These tropes recur in subsequent discussions of the surgical treatment of aphasia. In a 1911 paper the Russian surgeon, Ludwig M. Pussep (1875–1942) insisted that when dealing with operative intervention in such cases "theories of the localization of aphasia are naturally of immense importance."[28] Precise localization of function had placed neurosurgery on a scientific foundation. But Pussep also reiterated the tenet that a synergic relationship existed between theory and practice. Every operation on the brain had to be viewed "not only purely with a view to helping the patient, but also from the standpoint of the physiology of the nervous system, that is, from the purely scientific standpoint."[29] He thus felt obligated to state his compliance with and allegiance to the moral imperatives of scientific medicine.

The interplay between therapeutic and cognitive interests was especially evident in the matter of theory choice. Pussep referred to Pierre Marie's attempt to overturn existing localization theory by declaring that the true seat of the lesion causing motor aphasia lay in the subcortical ganglia, not in "Broca's region" (see chapter 6). Other authors, Pussep noted, had resisted this attempt to redraw the received map of cerebral function. Practical issues depended upon the outcome of this dispute between authorities: if Broca's theory was upheld, "indications for surgery are at our disposal [*vorhanden*], and these are entirely clear and comprehensible; but if Marie's theory is deemed valid then operative intervention, in the absence of obvious indications and urgency, is hardly ever an option."[30]

The surgeon had a clear interest in seeing Broca's doctrine vindicated. Intervention to remedy an affection of a cortical region of the brain was a realistic and "logical" option. If, however, Marie's theory was correct then surgical attempts to cure aphasia lost their rationale; they were de-

---

[26] Ibid., p. 306.

[27] Ibid.

[28] L. M. Pussep, "Operative Behandlung der traumatische Aphasien," *Journal für Psychologie und Neurologie* 17 (1911): 201–14, p. 203.

[29] Ibid., p. 201.

[30] Ibid., p. 203.

prived of their "point" [*Zweckmässigkeit*].[31] Pussep's argument may also be seen as a particular instance of the general surgical bias in favour of the precise localization of pathogenic lesions and against more constitutional or holist conceptions of disease.

The results of previous attempts to relieve motor aphasia by means of surgery could help to resolve this theoretical issue. A survey of the literature revealed, Pussep maintained, that operations to relieve pressure on Broca's region had led to an "almost complete restoration of speech." These facts, as well as his own experience, convinced Pussep of "the presence of a speech centre in Broca's gyrus, and operative intervention must have as its purpose gaining access [*Erreichung*] to this centre."[32] Surgical experience thus helped resolve the theoretical issue.

To a far greater extent than Macewen, Pussep's text recognized that even if the theory of cerebral localization was well grounded, and even if this knowledge was applied judiciously in a particular case, a further translation process must occur. When the skull remained intact the question arose of how the surgeon was to determine the position of Broca's gyrus before commencing his operation. Between the 1880s and the second decade of the twentieth century a variety of more or less complicated devices had been contrived to enable the surgeon to penetrate the opacity of the skull virtually before he essayed to do so actually.

Pussep himself favoured the more simple of these technologies, which, if not as precise as some of the instruments then available, "suffices for the demands of practical brain surgery." By drawing two lines on the patient's head orientated to certain of the bones of the skull, it was, he claimed, possible to ascertain the location of the speech and motor centers with tolerable accuracy. On occasion, however, even when the brain had been exposed to view, the identity of the "speech center" was not obvious. In such cases, Pussep maintained that electrical stimulation—a technique borrowed from the physiologist—could serve "to localize the parts of the cortex that control speech."[33]

Pussep's account revealed, however, almost by way of an aside just how tenuous was the relation between the graphic clarity of the maps and diagrams that adorned physiological texts and the reality confronting the surgeon in the exigent circumstances of an operation. The localization of the gyri, he remarked, "is far from constant and, moreover, often altered by pathological processes."[34] In other words, it was sometimes difficult for the surgeon to discern the sites that theory indicated he should target.

[31] Ibid., pp. 203–4.
[32] Ibid., p. 204.
[33] Ibid., pp. 206–7.
[34] Ibid., p. 207.

Despite the light cast by the labors of physiologists, navigating the intracranial territory in which the surgeon had to work therefore remained a fraught, sometimes desperate, enterprise.

The case histories with which Pussep concluded his paper revealed, however, the worth of grappling with the manifold difficulties facing the brain surgeon. His labors did more than add to the stock of scientific knowledge; they could give real relief to the patient. There was no perceived tension between these dual endeavors. After surgery, Pussep noted, one previously almost completely aphasic patient began "already towards evening spontaneously to enunciate words much more clearly and fluently." Subsequently, "his speech improved more and more each day."[35]

There is an evident delight and pride in this observation of the patient's progress which is also found in other accounts of the results of surgical intervention. Some accounts of the improvement achieved verge on the lyrical. Zachary Cope in 1914 reported that:

> Recovery of speech after the operation was exceedingly quick. The next day the patient asked for some dinner, and in general showed a marvellous improvement. Within a week all her disabilities were removed, and instead of the stolid, non-comprehending countenance was the intelligent, mobile face, readily smiling and appreciating every remark made to her.[36]

Here the surgeon had done no less than restore the personality of the patient.

The neurosurgical literature acknowledged, however, that even successful interventions sometimes failed to produce a total remission of symptoms. Moreover, in many cases of aphasia surgery was not indicated. Other forms of treatment had therefore to be pursued. Instead of the dramatic, almost instantaneous results obtained by means of an operation, these alternative strategies involved a prolonged and arduous interaction between patient and practitioner. And, rather than saltatory leaps, the most that could be expected of such therapeutic regimens was a series of hard-won incremental improvements in the patient's condition.

Talking Cures

The last two decades of the nineteenth century saw, especially in the German-speaking world, a burgeoning literature on the treatment of language disorders in general. Aphasia received its share of attention in these texts. After a lull, there was renewed interest during and after the First World

---

[35] Ibid., p. 210.
[36] V. Zachary Cope, "Notes of a Case of Traumatic Sensory Aphasia, Treated Successfully by Trephining and Removal of Clot," *Proceedings of the Royal Society of Medicine* 7 (1914): 128–30, p. 130.

War when neurologists were faced with the task of treating large numbers of brain damaged soldiers.

This literature acknowledged that some more or less successful methods of treating aphasia had been found in the past. These techniques had, however, been employed empirically or been stumbled upon by good fortune.[37] Often they were simply borrowed from the standard routines used to teach language skills to deaf and dumb, retarded, as well as "normal" children. While such borrowing was to a degree legitimate and even inevitable, Fritz Mohr in 1905 warned against too facile a transfer of methods appropriate to these other fields of pedagogy to the treatment of the aphasic.[38] The desideratum was the creation of a *systematic* approach to the treatment of aphasia in place of the ad hoc regimes that had prevailed before.

The widely held assumption that techniques developed in other disciplinary spheres were appropriate to the "education" of the aphasic is, however, symptomatic of a theme pervading the literature: namely, that there was a close analogy between the condition of aphasia and the state of childhood.[39] Although writers like Mohr were sometimes anxious to qualify this comparison, the aphasic/child couplet was so deeply embedded in the literature as to be ineradicable. This equation of the aphasic with the infantile is, incidentally, indicative of the importance ascribed to linguistic competence in received notions of the fully formed individual.

On this analogy the doctor occupied in relation to his patient something of the place of a schoolteacher or a parent. Thus Charles Mills wrote that: "The education of the sensory aphasic is that of a child. An object is held in front of him, the name is told, a picture is shown, and the word is pronounced, spelled and written." While in the case of a patient suffering from motor aphasia, he noted that:

> we adopted what may be called the 'Mother's Method.' Beginning with the labials, we taught him to say *papa, apap, appa.* . . . Then we taught him to say *baba, abab, abba*; then *mama, amam, amma*; then *wee wee*; and so on throughout the alphabet.[40]

---

[37] See, for instance, Bastian, *Treatise*, p. 352. For a general account of methods of aphasia therapy since the nineteenth century see: David Howard and Frances M. Hatfield, *Aphasia Therapy: Historical and Contemporary Issues* (London: Lawrence Erlbaum, 1987), pp. 16–57.

[38] Mohr, "Zur Behandlung," p. 1013.

[39] The notion that the speechless man was childlike predates the beginnings of the aphasia literature proper. In 1812 D. J. Larrey wrote of one brain-damaged patient: "he formed a new language for himself, in the same way that children do when they begin to babble." *Mémoires de chirurgie militaire, et campagnes*, 4 vols. (Paris: J. Smith, 1812–17), vol. 3, p. 322.

[40] Charles K. Mills, "Treatment of Aphasia by Training," *Journal of the American Medical Association* 43 (1904): 1939–49, p. 1944.

It is worth noting that in this instance the physician(s) explicitly assumes the nurturing role of the *female* parent.

In a similar vein the London neurologist Samuel Alexander Kinneir Wilson (1878–1937) in 1915 declared that: "In all cases, the method [of treating aphasics] is essentially one of imitating the procedures by which a child first learns the elements of speech."[41] One advantage of this analogy was that it rendered relevant to aphasia therapy the considerable body of theory on child psychology and education that had been developed in the course of the nineteenth century.

Those who at the turn of the twentieth century sought to limn a systematic program for re-educating aphasics were concerned to purge treatment of its "empirical" character; a recurring theme was the need to begin all discussions of therapy with a review of the current theoretical understanding of how language was represented in the brain and how it might be impaired by illness or injury. Matters were somewhat complicated by the fact that there was a notable lack of agreement on at least some aspects of this subject. Kinnier Wilson in 1913 noted that: "Round the subject of aphasia recent discussion has raged with an intensity that one had almost thought was foreign to any scientific study." He maintained nonetheless that there was a body of "classical views which have been built up by the labors of half a century" that could serve as a foundation for approaching the condition.[42]

There is a parallel here with the neurosurgeon's insistence that effective intervention in cases of aphasia depended upon the existence of reliable maps of the brain that in turn derived from the growth of physiological knowledge. In the case of nonsurgical treatment, however, the manner in which theory was to be translated into practice was less obvious. Physicians did not act upon the brain directly; but they did use the received accounts of the workings of the cerebral apparatus to generate narratives explanatory of their own practice.

Thus a common locution was that aphasia therapy was a matter of re-educating the "language centers." It was the patient's brain that was the true focus of therapeutic effort. The theory of compensation explained how damage to these centers and their internuncial links might be remedied. The activity of dormant centers on the opposite side of the brain might be aroused or new pathways established in the dominant hemisphere to replace those that had been lost. Techniques were then sought to put these principles into action. One way to excite the subordinate

---

[41] Kinnier Wilson, "Treatment," p. 697.

[42] S. A. Kinnier Wilson, "Treatment of Disorders of Expression (Aphasia, Apraxia, etc.)," in William A. White and Smith Ely Jelliffe (eds.), *The Modern Treatment of Nervous and Mental Diseases*, 2 vols. (London: Henry Kimpton, 1913), 475–504, pp. 475–76.

hemisphere into action was by encouraging the patient to try to write with his left hand. The rationale for this practice rested on the theory that:

> the development of the speech coordination centre in the left hemisphere is directly connected with righthandedness in man. When the left speech centre is destroyed it is appropriate to try to educate the right hemisphere to compensate. Writing exercises with the left hand should promote and support this by prompting the right hemisphere to perform more refined actions and at the same time . . . also forming association pathways between the written word [*Schriftbild*] and sound sequence in the right hemisphere.[43]

Localization theory thus allowed physicians a means to *account* for their actions.

Damaged language centers and pathways could also be replaced or rebuilt by means of a variety of other techniques. The overwhelming emphasis was upon the central role of *exercise* in restoring brain function; the cerebral centers were depicted as akin to muscles the activity of which could be enhanced by repeated use. Speech therapy was, in effect, a form of physiotherapy. Indeed German texts advocated a system *Gehirngymnastik* to "train" the cerebral centers to perform at new levels of efficiency.[44] The use of this term may reflect the growing enthusiasm in the late nineteenth century for athletic pursuits as a valuable complement to and stimulant of intellectual activity, as well as a general somatic bias.[45]

The kind of brain gymnastics recommended resembled muscular training in several respects. It involved the prolonged repetition of certain exercises designed to enhance the performance of the language centers; above all, great stress was laid upon the patient repeating long series of sounds at the doctor's direction. The simpler the sound the better: meaningless syllables were to be preferred to words. According to a proponent of this method, "One must . . . commence with the elements of speech and systematically practice individual sounds."[46]

The process of building or rebuilding the capabilities of the cerebral organs was thus conceived as a purely mechanical process: indeed, one

[43] A. Goldscheider, "Physiklische Therapie der Aphasie," in A. Goldscheider and Paul Jacob, *Handbuch der physikalischen Therapie*, 4 vols. (Leipzig: Georg Thieme, 1901–2), part 2, vol. 2, 537–552, p. 542.

[44] See: Emil Fröschels, "Ueber die Behandlung der Aphasie," *Archiv für Psychiatrie und Nervenkrankheiten* 53 (1914): 221–61, p. 250.

[45] For a discussion of this development see: Andrew Warwick, "Exercising the Student Body: Mathematics and Athleticism in Victorian Cambridge," in Christopher Lawrence and Steven Shapin (eds.), *Science Incarnate: Historical Embodiments of Natural Knowledge* (Chicago: Chicago University Press, 1998), pp. 288–326.

[46] H. Gutzmann, "Heilungsversuche bei centromotorischer und centrosensorischer Aphasie," *Archiv für Psychiatrie und Nervenkrankheiten* 28 (1896): 354–78, p. 358.

author recommended the use of a "reading machine" as a therapeutic aid. This consisted of a series of cases containing a row of letters that could be moved about a larger tray. The "teacher" would pull out letters one at a time so as gradually to form a word which the "pupil" [*Schüler*] would be obliged to read out without hesitation. Because the pupil did not know which letter was to come next nor what word would eventually appear on the board, he or she was forced to concentrate his attention on the individual components of the word.[47]

The aim of such exercises was to improve the pupil's fluency in articulating words; the semantic content of the patient's utterances, at least in the early stages of treatment, was deemed of little relevance. Indeed, the elimination of significance from what was said was often seen as essential to the success of a course of treatment; such considerations of meaning were likely to distract the patient from the true object of the exercise. An associated goal of these constant repetitions was to eliminate "false" memories—isolated remnants of the patient's previous speech patterns—that now hindered the acquisition of new speech skills.

The patient's role in this process was portrayed as passive and receptive. While the doctor acted, the aphasic merely reacted; moreover, this process of action and reaction was focussed upon the patient's body rather than on the mind. He or she spent much time simply imitating the doctor's sounds and seeking to mimic the mouth and tongue movements necessary to produce these phonemes. He or she would then seek to reproduce the sounds and movements in private using a mirror—"an important aid to self-control"[48]—to monitor bodily performance.

A marked agonistic theme runs through this narrative of recovery. There is, on the one hand, the patient's struggle with his or her own recalcitrant body. But there is also an additional element of conflict between patient and doctor. It was assumed that, left to follow his or her own inclinations, the patient would not recover, or at best the recovery would be seriously impaired. In order to achieve the best results, the patient had to be disciplined by the practitioner and compelled to conform to a tedious, exhausting regime. As in athletics, attainment of the desired skills depended on the presence of an exacting coach.[49] The ultimate goal

---

[47] Mohr, "Zur Behandlung," p. 1028.

[48] Gutzmann, "Heilungsversuche," p. 358.

[49] The analogy with other forms of "gymnastics" is again informative—especially when the imputed analogy between aphasic and child is recalled. Roberta J. Park has noted the tendency by the early 1900s to insist that children's play must be overseen by some adult expert and governed by a particular "training regime" if it was to attain the desired formative effects: "Biological Thought, Athletics, and the Formation of a 'Man of Character': 1830–1900," in J. A.. Mangan and James Walvin (eds.), *Manliness and Morality: Middle-Class Masculinity in Britain and America, 1800–1940* (Oxford: Manchester University Press, 1987), pp. 7–34, esp. pp. 17–18.

was, however, to replace this external supervision with an internalized surveillance by the patient of his or her linguistic performances. The degree
of success a therapeutic regime could ultimately achieve thus in large part
depended upon the doctor's ability to enlist the cooperation and to ensure
the perseverence of the patient.[50]

A multiplicity of technologies were devised to aid in the treatment of
aphasics according to these principles. Extensive use was made, for instance, of pictorial materials of different kinds to assist the patient in rebuilding associations between visual images and words. At their simplest
these comprised such tools as children's picture books in which word and
image were juxtaposed. More sophisticated materials specifically adapted
to therapeutic needs were also generated.[51] All these technologies were,
Gutzmann insisted, means to a single end: "The creation and exercise of
a new motor speech centre."[52]

Sensory aphasia was, it was generally conceded, more difficult to treat,
and required a different repertoire of methods. Gutzmann himself favored
the use of comprehension exercises similar to those used in teaching children to read.[53] The rationale for these operations was again to act indi-
rectly on an imagined brain surface where dormant sensory language centers waited to be discovered and developed.

After 1900, however, there was a tendency to question the adequacy of
this "anatomical" conception of the nature and goals of therapy. This
formed part of the wider critique of the received understanding of the
subject. While the old regime and its methods were not discarded, there
were calls for a more "psychological" approach to the task of treating the
aphasic. Kinnier Wilson in 1913 insisted that: "a given aphasic symptom-
complex can be looked at in two ways: what is the site of the lesion producing the symptoms, and what is the nature of the physiological or psychical
disturbance produced?" Each case of aphasia was thus "double-sided" and
this had to be reflected in its treatment—"for that may be directed either
to the improvement of the anatomical or rather pathological substratum,
or of the psycho-physiological disturbance, and in each instance the fashion of the treatment differs widely from the other."[54] Experience in the
treatment of war neuroses was supposed to have provided a model for what
could be achieved by attending to the patient's mind as well as to the
body. These disorders had originally been considered somatic in nature—
as the results of a physical "shell shock." Later, however, they were classi-

---

[50] Gutzmann, "Heilungsversuche," p. 378.
[51] For a typical summary of the various techniques employed see: Emil Fröschels, *Sprach-
und Stimmstörungen (Stammeln, Stottern usw.)* (Wien: Julius Springer, 1929), pp. 19–22.
[52] Gutzmann, "Heilungsversuche," p. 363.
[53] Ibid., pp. 365–67.
[54] Kinnier Wilson, "Treatment," p. 476.

fied as psychological reactions to the emotional traumas of war to be treated by various forms of verbal and suggestive therapy.[55]

Mohr, who had himself been active in treating neurotics during the war,[56] in 1925 maintained that an inversion of this sequence was possible: numerous disorders of the nervous system that *were* the results of physical injury nonetheless presented a significant mental component to which therapeutic attention must also be directed.[57] In all cases of aphasia, whatever the underlying brain lesion, the "psychic side" of the disorder was not to be underestimated.[58]

One consequence of this reorientation towards the psychological was that the literature increasingly came to insist on the need to individualize therapy—a point upon which advocates of a psychological approach to war neuroses had insisted. Physicians dealing with aphasics also came to insist that in framing their treatment they had to take account of the distinct, possibly unique, "personalities" of patients. In the therapeutic relationship the doctor was therefore as much concerned with the restoration of a person as with rebuilding the networks of a theorized brain. If the basis of the earlier therapeutic regime had been an analogy with the relation between athlete and coach, or perhaps between mother and infant, the new model much more resembled that of an interaction between equals—even though one party was, for reasons beyond his or her control, deprived of the full exercise of their normal faculties. Eliasberg accordingly praised a colleague who had achieved remarkable results in a particular case because: "He laboured not only at [the patient's] speech impairments, but also on his total personality."[59]

Eliasberg remarked upon how the therapeutic regime in this instance had been carefully tailored to the contours of this individuality. While conventional methods, such as the repetition of meaningless syllables, had been employed, these techniques had been effective because they conformed with the patient's inclinations and aptitudes. In a diagnostic protocol Eliasberg maintained that among the topics that must be explored

[55] On the shell shock phenomenon see: Paul Frederick Lerner, *Hysterical Men: War, Neurosis and German Mental Medicine, 1914–1921*, Columbia University PhD., 1996; Elaine Showalter, *The Female Malady: Women, Madness and English Culture, 1830–1980* (London: Virago Press, 1985), chapter 7; Martin Stone, "Shell-Shock and the Psychologists," in W. F. Bynum, Roy Porter and Michael Shepard, *The Anatomy of Madness*, 2 vols. (London: Tavistock, 1985), pp. 242–271; Allan Young, *The Harmony of Illusions: Inventing Post-Traumatic Stress Disorder* (Princeton: Princeton University Press, 1995), chapter 2.

[56] Fritz Mohr, "Aus der Praxis der Psychotherapie," *Medizinisches Klinik* 13 (1917): 1116–19; "Die Behandlung der Kriegsneurosen," *Therapeutische Monatschrift* 30 (1916): 131–41; "Grundsätzliches zur Kriegsneurosenfrage," *Med. Klinik* 12 (1916): 90–93.

[57] Mohr, *Psychophysische Behandlungen*, p. ix.

[58] Ibid., p. 75.

[59] Eliasberg, "Die Praxis," p. 238.

in each case of aphasia was the patient's "general personality type before and after the illness. Its mode of thought, its educational type."[60]

The literature in general reiterated this need to adapt treatment to the patient's "personality." In Mohr's words, "individualization . . . is the *conditio sine qua non* of every success in the treatment of aphasia." By "individualization" he meant classification of the patient according to some more or less elaborate psychological schema. In particular, some version of Charcot's distinction between "auditive," "visual," and "motor" types was of special relevance when planning how to approach any particular case.[61]

It was also necessary to classify the patient according to his or her *social* type. The "orator," he declared, had different linguistic needs than the businessman; and such considerations had to be taken into account when planning treatment.[62] A patient's class as well as status was of importance when establishing priorities and evaluating results. The therapist should bear in mind:

> how primitive is the speech of common people [*einfachen Mannes*], especially in respect of sentence formation, when compared to that of the educated: on these grounds, there is no reason for us to make any special effort to correct agrammatism when dealing with the majority of aphasics from the lower classes.[63]

In other words, this particular form of aphasia, in which the ability to construct coherent propositions was impaired, was a significant disability only among certain strata of society; that is, among those who were allowed to have something to say.

Class was also relevant to prognosis. An American neurologist remarked in 1904 of how different patients attained very variable degrees of recovery from similar insults to the nervous system. This was, in part, a question of personality: "A man of intelligence or education, or of both, and especially if he is endowed with a strong character, will often advance with great rapidity on the road to recovery." The level of medical care that an aphasic could afford was, however, also relevant. Mills invited his medical reader

> to recall and compare his hospital experience with his experience in private practice to appreciate the full force of these statements. In the nervous wards of the Philadelphia Hospital, where a number of aphasics of different types are always to be found, the majority of the patients have little or no education.

[60] Ibid., p. 235.
[61] Mohr, "Zur Behandlung," p. 1015.
[62] Ibid., pp. 1014–15.
[63] Ibid., p. 1029.

Among these patients recoveries from aphasia are comparatively rare and are relatively incomplete, while better cared for patients show much greater improvement and approach more nearly to complete recovery when properly and persistently trained.[64]

There is no suggestion here that the hospital patients were inherently less capable of recovery; merely a frank recognition that the degree of improvement varied directly with an individual's ability to purchase dedicated medical attention.

Mills, like Mohr, held that therapy should seek to restore to the patient the language appropriate to his or her background. There was "a grammar of the slums. If a child who lives in the Bowery and uses the language of Jimmie Fadden becomes aphasic, he must regain this particular sort of language."[65] Notions of what constituted normality and health therefore varied with a patient's social class and status; an implicit and sometimes explicit goal of therapy was to respect and maintain those distinctions. The rhetorical insistence on the need to respect individuality notwithstanding, each social station was deemed to have its own appropriate form of personality.

Conclusion

Considerations of class and occupation were not entirely absent from the main body of the aphasia archive (see chapter 3). It is nonetheless the case that the patient is a far more nuanced figure in the therapeutic appendix to this literature, at least in its later "psychological" phase.[66] Instead of merely being a receptacle for a diseased brain, he or she is allowed a social situation, biography, personal traits, a circle of friends and family—and even, on occasion, a will. All these details are, moreover, deemed relevant to the conduct of and prospects for therapy. In the case of the post-1914 literature there is even a sense of the patient's, and physician's, place in a wider historical setting.

Moreover, while in most of the aphasia literature the aphasic is a passive object revolving haplessly in the clinical gaze, when it came to therapy he was to some degree allowed an active role; authors conceded that success depended upon the doctor's ability to recruit the patient as an active part-

[64] Mills, "Treatment," p. 1945.
[65] Ibid., p. 1949.
[66] Henry Head's case histories (chapter 5) form an exception to this generalization. Although he was not particularly concerned with treatment, Head's texts do show the same concerns with personality and class that figure in the therapeutic literature.

ner in his treatment. The two were locked together in an intense, often protracted and sometimes even intimate relationship. It was commonplace by the end of the nineteenth century for the doctor to lay hands on his patient; the aphasic was unusual in that on occasion his treatment even involved touching the physician.[67]

Various otherwise shadowy or even invisible figures also appear in these accounts as active agents: not only doctor and patient, but also friends, family, and nurses figure as actors in the drama of recovery. Emil Fröschels, in particular, stressed the role of such allies in his efforts to relieve the aphasia of wounded soldiers who came under his care. He even named one of the nurses who had assisted in therapy. Other patients were also recruited to play a part in treatment. Moreover, Fröschels strived to make his aphasic patients sufficiently independent of his help so that after they had left the clinic they could pursue their treatment themselves.[68]

A different image of the clinician is also projected by these texts. Chapter 1 noted a tendency in the classic aphasiological narrative for the author virtually to erase himself qua individual from his account. The true narrator was less some concrete historical individual than an ideal scientific observer shorn of historical contingencies. The orientation of this depersonalized observer to the sick and injured individuals that passed through his gaze was one of pure curiosity uncontaminated by any other interest. The stance is thus one of a carefully constructed objectivity. The patient is considered purely as an object of scientific inquiry. At the same time, the cognitive interest of the observer is dissociated from all other possible modes of knowing and responding to the aphasic. In the therapeutic literature there is, on the other hand, some mitigation of this austerity and singleness of purpose.

Eliasberg began his discussion of aphasia therapy by posing two questions to his professional colleagues: "1. Should we treat aphasics? 2. Can we treat aphasics?"[69] The latter was a technical matter; there were, as we have seen, resources that could be mobilized to relieve the aphasic condition. These techniques, however, made extreme demands on the time, perseverance, and skill of the medical practitioner; in this respect aphasia therapy was similar to the other equally labour-intensive talking cure, psychoanalysis.[70] The real question was therefore whether the aphasic de-

---

[67] Fröschels, "Ueber die Behandlung," pp. 233, 237.

[68] "Offizielles Protokoll der k. k. Gesellschaft der Aertze in Wien," *Wiener klinische Wochenschrift* 27 (1914): 1650.

[69] Eliasberg, "Die Praxis," p. 234.

[70] Josef Breuer spent several hours a day with the classic hysteric Anna O, whose symptoms included an inability to speak in her native German although she could still communicate in English.

served such attention from his medical attendant. In order to convince his readers that these patients did merit this level of expenditure of medical energy, Eliasberg invited them to *empathize* with the aphasic:

> Let us imagine the condition of an adult robbed of the full possession of speech through illness. It is truly terrible. If the motor functions are chiefly impaired, the patient hears, sees, comprehends and yet cannot communicate with those around him. The enormous irritability, the outbursts of rage, the fits of weeping of these patients need not be taken for symptoms of arteriosclerosis of the brain. They are an understandable response by the patient to his predicament.[71]

Among other things, this passage goes some way to *de*-pathologize the aphasic: to show him or her to be a normal human being reacting to extraordinary circumstances in an understandable way.

The plight of the sensory aphasic was also tragic; the condition might easily be mistaken by friends and family for insanity. In truth intelligence was not impaired and the patient was aware of these false perceptions; this made the predicament of those afflicted with this form of aphasia all the more poignant. Conscious of his or her state, the patient was anxious to break free from it and sought the means to communicate. Anyone who helped the aphasic again become a competent social actor would earn the gratitude both of the patient and of relatives.[72] The aphasic was thus represented in ways designed to provoke an active compassion; this was a subjective, humanitarian rather than a purely scientific view of the patient.[73] The reader was invited to share an affective response to the predicament of the speechless man or woman; the resulting compassion would prompt him to seek to *alleviate* that condition.

Those practitioners who undertook this mission faced a daunting task: aphasia therapy, Mohr declared, "will always be among the more difficult branches of medical endeavour."[74] This difficulty was, however, presented as a challenge that would further incite the enthusiasm of the dedicated clinician. Treating aphasics was "for the doctor no easy undertaking, but often a truly gratifying one."[75] Stern similarly wrote of speech therapy as among the most "fruitful and beneficent" fields of medical endeavor.[76]

---

[71] Ibid. This appeal for empathy from the reader is reminiscent to that made by Lordat when describing his own plight as an aphasic: see chapter 1.

[72] Ibid., p. 235.

[73] Cf. Thomas W. Laqueur, "Bodies, Details, and the Humanitarian Narrative," in Lynn Hunt (ed.), *The New Cultural History* (Berkeley: University of California Press, 1989), pp. 176–204.

[74] Mohr, "Zur Behandlung," p. 1015.

[75] Ibid., p. 1068.

[76] Stern, "Die Grundprinzipien," p. 247.

Fröschels provided a personal testimony to the same effect when he concluded a case report with the proud boast that after two months of treatment, "I succeeded in curing the patient's speech disorder."[77]

A different set of medical values to those predominant elsewhere in the aphasia canon is thus inscribed in these texts. In many ways they represent a more traditional, humanistic notion of the physician in which medical activity is validated by reference to the relief of human suffering it can achieve. The physician's primary responsiblity on this model is to his patient; achievement is measured by his skill in returning to health the sick man or woman. The clinician's intellect is chiefly exercised with seeking ingenious and effective means to relieve an affliction. Mohr, for instance, detailed how he exercised his aphasics' diminished language skills by asking them to translate prose into poetry and vice versa; riddles and jokes could also serve to sharpen the patient's linguistic skills.[78] Even in this therapeutic literature, however, the medical man's responsibility to science is never altogether forgotten; at the same time as he treats the patient he still remains alert to any appearances that might cast light on the nature of aphasic disorders or on the normal workings of the brain.

Moreover, even when the focus was chiefly therapeutic, the rationale for attempts to relieve the aphasic did not have to take the form of an appeal to humanitarian sentiments. By the end of the period with which this book deals other repertoires of values were available within which to frame the cure of brain-damaged patients. Both postures were represented in Kurt Goldstein's (1878–1965) *Die Behandlung, Fürsorge und Begutachtung der Hirnverletzungen* (*The Treatment, Care and Assessment of Brain Injuries*) published in 1919.

The book is an account of the regime at a hospital [*Lazarett*] in Frankfurt directed by Goldstein specializing in the treatment of soldiers suffering from brain injuries, many of whom included language impairments among their symptoms.[79] In his account of the methods employed in this institution Goldstein rehearsed many of the themes we have already seen in the early twentieth-century therapeutic literature. He insisted, for instance, on the need to individualize treatment after exhaustive investigations had revealed the exact nature of a patient's disabilities.[80] He also

---

[77] Fröschels, "Ueber die Behandlung," p. 246.

[78] Mohr, "Zur Behandlung," pp. 1045, 1061.

[79] On the founding of the Frankfurt *Lazarett* see: Anne Harrington, *Reenchanted Science: Holism in German Culture from Wilhelm II to Hitler* (Princeton: Princeton University Press, 1996), pp. 145–46.

[80] Goldstein, *Die Behandlung, Fürsorge und Begutachtung der Hirnverletzungen: Zugleich ein Beitrag zur Verwendung psychologischer Methoden in der Klinik* (Leipzig: F.C.W. Vogel, 1919), pp. 68–69.

stressed the need to adapt treatment to the "whole personality" of the patient; this included his "intelligence, education, [and] experience [*Anschauungskreis*]."[81]

But there were also significant differences between this account and typical discussions of treatment in the earlier literature. First, Goldstein's is a description of the therapeutic efforts of an *institution* rather than of a single medical practitioner. The needs of the patient were addressed by a collective of therapists, not all of whom were medically qualifed, rather than by the solitary physician who predominates elsewhere in the literature. Goldstein insisted in particular that the strictly medical and the "social"—that is, the rehabilitative and retraining—sides of treatment should not be separated; the two went "hand in hand."[82]

Goldstein provided a map of the hospital indicating the various departments engaged in its cooperative effort. As well as the hospital building itself there were units devoted to the psychological assessment of patients and to their reeducation and retraining.[83] The former facilities were of special importance to the workings of the institution: these laboratories provided the means for "fruitful collaboration between doctor and psychologist." The thorough psychological evaluation of the patient by these specialists formed the basis for the program of treatment pursued in a given case.[84]

Such multiplication of the personnel involved in therapy might seem likely to diminish the intensity of the patient-doctor relationship described elsewhere in the literature. Moreover, an acknowledgement of the vital, rather than ancillary, function played in the process by those without medical qualfications appears to detract from the central role of the physician. These tendencies are, however, quickly counteracted. The number of personnel at work in the hospital made imperative "a constant, intimate *collaboration of all involved under a leader*. This role naturally falls upon the physician in charge of the hospital." There was thus a need for "continuous medical surveillance." This control might be secured by a medical presence at examinations. The doctor's attendance would, among other things, assure the patient's consent to investigative procedures at which he might otherwise balk because these would be perceived as somehow linked to therapy. But control could also be exercised by means of appropriate documentation. Lay personnel received precise written, as well as oral, instructions on how to complete the protocols entrusted to them.[85]

[81] Ibid., p. 137.

[82] Ibid., p. 1.

[83] Ibid., p. 3.

[84] Ibid., p. 73.

[85] Ibid., pp. 4, 219.

In the clinical setting itself the ideal was a continual personal supervision of each case by the medical director himself.[86] Given the number of patients and the complexity of the regime this was not practicable; much of the day-to-day treatment had to be delegated to junior staff. This lack of personal control could, however, be offset by means of paper chains. Goldstein described and reproduced in an appendix the "schemata" that were used to ensure uniformity in the evaluation of patients in the hospital regardless of the identity of the attending physician. These devices were designed to reduce as far as possible idiosyncrasy and to ensure uniformity in the results produced by different attendants. These documents were thus the descendants of the protocols for the examination of aphasics mentioned in chapter 3. The schedules established a series of routine tests designed to make possible at least a rough assessment of the patient's condition. When completed the forms were placed in the "hand of the Director," who scrutinized them in the company of their "issuers." This process of review by the senior physician was crucial to the proper use of these documents: "nothing would be more misleading than an uncritical employment of these schemata."[87]

Direct contact with the patient's body and performances was thus replaced by the perusal of a series of documents organized within a standard format. These included the results of various instrumental examinations which produced such graphic outcomes as curves "typical" of particular kinds of brain damage. The forms were conscientiously collated in files and entrusted to the care of a designated "official" [*Beamte*]. Any omissions in the completion of these protocols would be corrected retrospectively.[88]

Such technologies were designed to counteract the centrifugal tendencies inherent in the plurality of personnel at work in the clinic. By these means the director, though divorced from the routine work of the institution, maintained a kind of oversight over its operations. The basis for his decisions for the treatment and rehabilitation of a particular case was, however, chiefly derived from a knowledge of papers rather than of persons.

What Goldstein described was in effect a system of rational management. The institution he directed was quasi-bureaucratic in its division of labor and hierarchical organization. It employed officials as well as doctors and doctors who were in effect officials. The face-to-face relationship be-

---

[86] Compare the problems of coordinating the efforts of numerous subordinates confronted by Ivan Pavlov when he attempted to set up a physiological "factory." Through close personal supervision Pavlov was in this case able to ensure that his collaborators served in effect as extensions to his own senses. Daniel P. Todes, "Pavlov's Physiology Factory," *Isis* 88 (1997): 205–46.

[87] Goldstein, *Die Behandlung.*, p. 5.

[88] Ibid., p. 219.

tween a single authorial physician and "his" patient was effaced as a result of the necessity of processing large numbers of wounded men. The First World War was an industrial conflict that achieved a mass production of casualties; the facilities that dealt with this army of wounded had to be of a comparable order. The war, however, merely accelerated a trend toward more "scientific management" in the provision of health care that had been evident for some time.[89]

The war also left its mark on the therapeutic goals pursued in the hospital. The overriding purpose of military medicine during the conflict was to restore the wounded to a condition where they could again be of service, whether in the armed forces or as civilian workers.[90] Under this regime the interests of the individual were subordinate to those of the militant collective. In what otherwise reads like a humane and compassionate discussion of approaches to the treatment of war neuroses Mohr had insisted on the need to remind these patients of the need for "self-renunciation" and subordination to a cause greater than the individual ego.[91]

This collectivist ethos was in some ways antithetical to the patient-centered sentiments most characteristic of Goldstein's writings; it nonetheless found a place in his text. A key term in his diagnostic and therapeutic vocabulary is "competence" or "capacity" [*Leistungsfähigkeit*]. This denoted an individual's mental and physical capability to deal with his or her environment and followed from Goldstein's avowed "holistic" understanding of the operations of the normal and damaged brain.[92] One of the definitive characteristics of brain injury was that it impaired this capacity: it made the victim a less competent actor in the social and physical worlds. The various investigations that patients underwent in Goldstein's clinic were designed to identify the nature and extent of these deficits. The overriding goal of therapy was to seek to reverse this damage by restoring as far as possible lost abilities.

But while competence could be broadly construed as the totality of an individual's interactions with the environment, the overwhelming empha-

[89] Steve Sturdy and Roger Cooter have argued that in the Anglo-American context the rise of laboratory medicine occurred in the context of a broader process favorable to the ideals of scientific management. "Science, Scientific Management, and the Transformation of Medicine in Britain *c.* 1870–1950," *History of Science* 36 (1998): 421–66. See especially p. 429 for the move towards standardized record keeping and division of labor within the clinic.

[90] On this transformation see: Paul Lerner, "Rationalizing the Therapeutic Arsenal: German Neuropsychiatry in World War I," in Manfred Berg and Geoffrey Cocks (eds.), *Medicine and Modernity: Public Health and Medical Care in Nineteenth- and Twentieth-Century Germany* (Cambridge: Cambridge University Press, 1997), pp. 123, 129, 133–34.

[91] Mohr, "Behandlung der Kriegsneurosen," p. 136.

[92] See: Harrington, *Reenchanted Science*, pp. 146–48 for an account of the paradigmatic case in which these principles were first expounded.

sis in Goldstein's account is on capacity for *work* [*Arbeitsfähigkeit*]. The principal goal of the clinic was to reconstitute the patient as a productive laborer. The first page of the book proclaimed, "From the outset we must confront not only the question of: 'how do we secure the patient's health [and] existence,' but also: 'how do we make him, despite his impairments, again fit for work.' " This was an issue that arose with other forms of injury; but it was especially acute in the case of wounds to the brain because of the extent and duration of their consequences.[93] Once such issues were raised, the goal of therapy ceased to be merely to restore the wholeness of the individual; it was also to make him again of use to society rather than a burden on its resources. At the same time, however, the more starkly instrumental aspects of this imperative were tempered by the fact that capacity for work was central to the reconstitution of the patient as complete person while dependence on welfare was deemed detrimental to the patient's personality. Work was in a genuine sense deemed therapeutic.

The therapeutic appendix to the aphasiological canon undoubtedly possesses features that distinguish it from the rest of the literature. Patients emerge as objects of compassion with whom the physician enters into a close relationship in order to secure relief and recovery. After 1900, the "personality" of the aphasic becomes an object of much greater concern as do his or her social relations. There is, in short, something of a return to humanistic notions of medical practice as well as to a more concrete and complete conception of the patient. Goldstein's text, however, also shows other tendencies at work; it manifests evident tensions between divergent systems of values. The stress upon the special characteristics of the individual patient remains; but the object is to restore that individual, not only to personal wholeness, but also to a condition where he can serve the collective.

In a somewhat defensive passage in the conclusion of the book Goldstein acknowledged that by such purely utilitarian criteria the worth of the elaborate regime he had instituted in his establishment might be open to doubt. Some might say that the more lightly wounded soldiers with whom he dealt would have been able to return to a productive life without the assistance of this sophisticated evaluative and therapeutic regime. While in the more serious cases the economic benefits of such measures were incommensurable with the effort involved.[94] This was a tacit acknowledgment that, faced with a cost/benefit analysis, Goldstein's system might be found wanting.

In response Goldstein gestured to a more expansive notion of the medical role. Especially when dealing with head wounds the practitioner had

[93] Goldstein, *Die Behandlung*, p. 1.
[94] Ibid., p. 215.

to be motivated by more than "merely economic considerations." Even in cases where the physician could do next to nothing to improve the *Arbeitsfähigkeit* of a patient, "we are obliged on purely humanitarian grounds to do everything we can to allow the patient to make his life as tolerable as possible." Goldstein added, however, that happily this "wholly charitable point of view" was applicable in only a small number of instances. In the majority of cases the patient did indeed become "economically useful" [*wirtschaftlich leistungsfähig*] as a result of the treatment he had received. Goldstein pointed out, moreover, that after the war there would be such a shortage of fully competent workers in all professions that society would be obliged to make "the most economical use of the energies of those who are only partially fit for work [*mit den nur beschränkt arbeitsfähigen Kräften recht sparsam umzugehen*]."[95] The notions of health, humanity, and of the capacity to do socially useful work are thus inextricably intertwined. Humanist nostalgia had come to terms with the rigors of the modern.

[95] Ibid.

CONCLUSION

The human brain, a 3-pound mass of interwoven nerve cells
that controls our activity, is one of the most magnificent—
and mysterious—wonders of creation. The seat of human
intelligence, interpreter of senses, and controller of
movement, this incredible organ continues to intrigue
scientists and laymen alike.
(Presidential Proclamation 6158, 17 July 1990)

ADOLPH MEYER, an adoptive American neurologist, writing in the first decade of the twentieth century, allowed himself in his private jottings to muse upon the wider implications of the scientific endeavor in which he was engaged. Meyer posited a gulf between "the man who felt himself placed in and above nature . . . , and the man who felt himself heart and soul as part of nature, part of an orderly realm of objective facts and events." The transition between these two states of human consciousness was the achievement of nineteenth-century science; and within this movement, "no discovery was more fundamental than that of the so-called cerebral localization & the rise of the doctrine of aphasia & apraxia. Without it we might still be far from the objective psychology of to-day."[1] These discoveries were so crucial because the fact of a regular correlation between lesions of the third frontal convolution and impairment of speech was proof that the same *lawfulness* obtained in the workings of the mind as did in the material world. Meyer's words thus place the emergence of aphasiology firmly within the rise of an overarching scientific naturalism.

The crucial moment in the establishment of this naturalism is usually taken to be the foundation during the second half of the nineteenth century of the theory of evolution. At the center of this theory was the notion of the continuity that obtained within the living world; above all, evolution allowed for no qualitative distinction between humans and other animals. While some might concede that the structure of the human body showed clear affinities with that of other mammals, and, in particular, with that of primates, it was, however, still possible for those opposed to naturalism to make a stand on the issue of the distinctive nature of the human mind. Man might indeed be an animal; but he was a *rational* animal, a quality that elevated him above the rest of creation.

[1] Meyer Papers, Johns Hopkins University Archives, XIV/1/19.

The historic link between reason and the faculty of language was discussed in chapter 2. There I tried to show how the discovery of an organic seat for language posed a challenge for the assumption that the capacity of speech placed man above animals and mind above matter. For Meyer, writing after the existence of a material substrate for language had become an orthodoxy, it was simply a matter of fact that these once cherished distinctions could no longer be maintained. It is important to note, however, that even in the second half of the nineteenth century those intent on insisting on the special status of humanity still viewed language as a buttress against naturalism.

The philologist Max Müller was aware of the emergence of a new challenge to traditional metaphysics in the form of a neurologically based psychology, the forerunner of what came to be known as cognitive neuroscience. "Our mind," he declared,

> whether consisting of material impressions or intellectual concepts, was now to be submitted to the dissecting knife and the microscope. We were shown the nervous tubes, afferent and efferent, through which the shocks from without pass on to the sensitive and motive cells; the commissural tubes holding these cells together were laid bare before us; the exact place in the brain was pointed out where the messages were delivered; and it seemed as if nothing were wanting but a more powerful lens to enable us to see with our own eyes how, in the workshop of the brain, as in a photographic apparatus, the picture of the senses and the ideas of the intellect were being turned out in an endless variety.[2]

Modern imaging technology has, it might be argued, provided just such a "more powerful lens" to make visible the workings of the mind to the scientific gaze.

Müller determined to make a stand against the encroachment of scientific naturalism upon the realm of the human mind. In opposition to the tendency to collapse revered boundaries he insisted that there were "hard and fast lines in nature." He took it upon himself, in particular, "to warn the valiant disciples of Mr Darwin that before they can call man the descendant of a mute animal, they must lay a regular siege to a fortress of language which is not to be frightened into submission by a few random shots; the fortress of language, which, as yet, stands untaken and unshaken

---

[2] Max Müller, "Lectures on Mr Darwin's Philosophy of Language," *Fraser's Magazine* 7, 8ns (1873): 659–78; 1–24, 660. For a fuller account of Müller's dispute with Darwin see: Elizabeth Knoll, *Evolution and the Science of Language: Darwin, Müller, and Romanes on the Development of the Human Mind* (University of Chicago PhD Dissertation, 1987); idem, "The Science of Language and the Evolution of Mind," *Journal of the History of the Behavioural Sciences* 22 (1986): 3–22.

on the very frontier between the animal kingdom and man."[3] The detail of the martial metaphor is telling. Müller's defiance notwithstanding, it suggests that those intent on maintaining hard and fast lines between man and animal, spirit and matter, were a beleaguered force, forced on the defensive by the rampant hordes of naturalism. Among their last remaining strongholds was the bastion of language.

Müller had some acquaintance with the literature on aphasia; he referred in passing to Broca's claims of the localization of the seat of language as well as giving more detailed attention to John Hughlings Jackson's writings on the subject.[4] Indeed, Müller saw Jackson's distinction between rational and emotional language (see chapter 4) as a means of reinforcing categorical boundaries in nature. Animals did possess language, but only of the inferior, emotional kind. Human beings—especially "a man in a passion, or on a low scale of civilisation"[5]—also manifested this form of communication. What distinguished man was his superadded capacity for rational, or conceptual, language. The phenomena of aphasia, as detailed by Jackson, demonstrated that these two faculties were separable and thus independent. Darwin's contention that human speech had evolved from animal cries was thus refuted.[6]

Müller was fully prepared to concede that: "if a certain portion of the brain . . . happens to be affected by disease, the patient becomes unable to use the rational language; while, unless some other mental disease is added to aphasia, he retains the emotional language, and of communicating with others by means of signs and gestures." But, he added that,

> In saying this, I shall not be suspected, I hope, of admitting that the brain, or any part of the brain, secretes language as the liver secretes bile. My only object in referring to these medical observations and experiments was to show that the distinction between emotional and rational language is not artificial, or of a purely logical character, but is confirmed by the palpable evidence of the brain in its pathological affections.

[3] Ibid., p. 22.

[4] Darwin also alluded to the aphasia literature when trying to demonstrate the physical basis of language. "The intimate connection between the brain, as it is now developed in us, and the faculty of speech," he wrote, "is well shewn by those curious cases of brain-disease, in which speech is specially affected, as when the power to remember substantives is lost, whilst other words can be correctly used." *The Descent of Man, and Selection in Relation to Sex* [1871] (Princeton: Princeton University Press, 1981), part 1, p. 58.

[5] Müller, "Lectures," p. 677.

[6] Ibid., p. 675. On Darwin's views on the origins of language see: Robert J. Richards, *Darwin and the Emergence of Evolutionary Theories of Mind and Behavior* (Chicago: University of Chicago Press, 1987), chapter 5; Stephen G. Alter, *Darwinism and the Linguistic Image* (Baltimore: Johns Hopkins Press, 1998).

The brain, Müller insisted, was no more the seat of language than the eye the seat of the faculty of seeing:

> We cannot see without the eye, nor hear without the ear; perhaps we might say, we cannot speak without the 3rd convolution of the left anterior lobe of the brain; but neither can the eye see without us, the ear hear without us, the 3rd convolution of the brain speak without us. To look for the faculty of speech in the brain would, in fact, hardly be less Homeric than to look for the soul in the midriff.[7]

According to Müller, "no man of philosophical culture" would make the error of confusing the brain, a condition of the exercise of intellectual functions, with the seat of or cause of these functions. He tried to insist that there was a need to acknowledge something beyond the apparatus of the nervous system, an "I" or "we" to which agency must be ascribed. At the same time, however, Müller did not forego the opportunity to invoke the authority of "medical observations" when these seemed to bolster his case. The observations of John Hughlings Jackson might be deemed to characterize sound science as opposed to the groundless speculations of the Darwinians (Müller appeared oblivious to the evolutionary bent of Jackson's work). But an anxiety to find support for his distinctions in the "palpable evidence of the brain" is indicative of the power of the very icon that Müller's argument was supposed to subvert.

It is tempting to characterize such protests against the encroachment of naturalism in disciplinary terms: to see Müller as the representative of a traditional humanist understanding of language resisting the novel claims of natural science upon his domain. Such an interpretation would, however, be inadequate; there were those within the camp of science who shared similar misgivings over the tendency of the age. Frederic Bateman's contribution to the discourse of aphasia was discussed above (see chapter 3). He was undoubtedly an accredited player in that game. Nonetheless, Bateman expressed reservations similar to Müller's about the emerging conception of man's place in nature. He also shared Müller's conviction that language proved an insuperable stumbling block to naturalism. While

> conceding that Man, in his purely physical nature, is closely allied to certain members of the brute creation, I entirely repudiate the inference drawn from this analogy by Mr Darwin and other writers of the modern school of thought; for supposing it to be proved to a mathematical demonstration, that Man is like an Ape, bone for bone, muscle for muscle, nerve for nerve, what then? What does this prove, if it can be shown that Man possesses a *distinct attribute*, of which not a trace can be found in the Ape,—an attribute of such

---

[7] Ibid., p. 676.

a nature as to create an immeasurable gulf between the two? This attribute I assert to be the faculty of Articulate Language, which I maintain to be a difference, *not only of degree, but of kind.*[8]

Bateman, however, was not a representative scientific voice; his views possess a quaint, antique quality. Meyer came much closer to capturing the spirit of the modern age.

. . . . .

The epigraph to this Conclusion is taken from Proclamation 6158 issued on 17 July 1990 by George Bush, 41st President of the United States of America. The Proclamation followed from a joint resolution of both Houses of Congress that designated the 1990s as the "Decade of the Brain." This decision by organs of state to celebrate a bodily organ strikes at least some observers as incongruous. The incongruity proceeds from the assumption that holders of high government office do not normally concern themselves with anything as ignoble as the contents of a body cavity. It would, for instance, be inconceivable that President and Congress should proclaim a "Decade of the Spleen," or of the liver; such glorification of the lower body would simply be too carnivalesque. Clearly the brain is a very special viscus.

A close reading gives some hints as to why it might seem appropriate for statesmen to take a particular interest in the encephalon. They, after all, represent the head of the body politic: *their* functions of deliberation and direction parallel those ascribed to the cerebral mass. In a democracy, moreover, the executive and legislature are said to represent the members of the commonwealth just as the various parts of the body are represented on the cortex. By celebrating the brain they thus pay a compliment to themselves. It would be redundant to labor a metaphor that has been commonplace in Western culture for centuries, one that was, mutatis mutandis, familiar to Elizabeth I as well as to John Hughlings Jackson.[9] It is sufficient to note that "The Brain" in question is here invested with personality of a certain kind.

This encomium to the brain is the preamble to a call for further research into its mysterious workings with the aim of relieving the numerous maladies that occur when it is injured or diseased. These include "degenerative

---

[8] Frederic Bateman, *Darwinism Tested by Language* (London: Rivingtons, 1877), pp. 85–86.

[9] In the early-modern period, however, the head had still to contend for dominance with the heart; complete craniocentrism was the achievement of the nineteenth century. For an account of Renaissance analogies between body politic and body natural see: E. M. W. Tillyard, *The Elizabethan World Picture* (Harmondsworth: Penguin Books, 1976), pp. 101–6.

disorders such as Alzheimer's, as well as stroke, schizophrenia, autism, and impairments of speech, language, and hearing." For those suffering from such conditions there is cause for hope: "for a new era of discovery is dawning in brain research. Powerful microscopes, major strides in the study of genetics, and advances in brain imaging devices are giving physicians and scientists ever greater insight into the brain." As well as assisting those afflicted by brain disease such research "may also prove valuable in our war on drugs, as studies provide greater insight into how people become addicted to drugs and how drugs affect the brain."

Such utterances are indicative of the iconic status "The Brain" has assumed in our culture as the twentieth century draws to a close. To a remarkable extent, the brain is identified as the source of those attributes that are most definitive of ourselves; in the words of Joint Resolution 174, the brain is deemed to translate "neurophysiologic events into behavior, thought, and emotion." What was for Max Müller a "Homeric" solecism is today a commonplace. Scientific investigation into this organ is seen as the obvious means to protect those attributes, enhance human life, and to address social ills such as narcotics abuse.[10] Even presidents find it necessary to make obeisance to these twin idols. Humanitarian sentiment is openly coupled with the expectation that this branch of science will, as have so many others, yield potent weapons for the state to deploy in a particularly vexatious war. Moreover, research into neuroscience may also, according to the organizers of a series of symposia intended to mark the "Decade of the Brain," have "implications for American economic competitiveness."

The report goes on to enthuse: "If we are entering a second Enlightenment, its underlying science could well be neuroscience." Physics had, it is argued, been the intellectual underpinning of the first Enlightenment in the eighteenth century—"a period of intellectual revolution that spawned the idea of contemporary democracy." The original Enlightenment failed, however, because "it was unable to translate humanistic theory into practice and thereby improve the lot of all." A second, more comprehensive Enlightenment based upon neuroscience, on the other hand, "becomes more likely as we increase our understanding of how the brain works to create ideas, to learn about one another, to govern our interactions in society."[11] Neuroscience thus promises a way to the good life; potentially it furnishes the *techne* to create a new ideal Republic of which Plato could scarcely have dreamed.

---

[10] In February 1999 it was reported that a Russian neurosurgeon had pioneered an operation designed to cure heroin addicts of their dependency by ablating part of their brain.

[11] *Neuroscience, Memory, and Language. Volume I of Papers Presented at a Symposium Series. Executive Summary.* http://lcweb.loc.gov/loc/brain/summary.html

This book has sought to chronicle some of the early episodes in the making of the modern brain. Its theme has been how what was for centuries regarded as humanity's most definitive attribute became engrossed by the substance of the cerebral cortex and thus a proper object of natural scientific investigation. One theme of the book has been the way in which this investigation was made to seem mundane: as part of the work that medical practitioners routinely performed at the bedside of brain-damaged patients. At the same time, however, evidence has been presented to show an awareness of the portentous nature of the enterprise of establishing the material conditions of language. Paul Broca and his supporters in the Société d'Anthropologie could scarcely have predicted the awesome power that would be ascribed in the 1990s to the science they helped to found. But their words also display a faith that enhancing knowledge of the physiology of mind was at once a contribution to the enterprise of Enlightenment with all that implied for culture and society.

The "Decade of the Brain" was intended to "enhance public awareness of the benefits to be derived from brain research"; and to this end "appropriate programs, ceremonies, and activities" are enjoined.[12] The need to disseminate scientific understanding among the populace is another Enlightenment imperative: a citizenry educated in the facts of nature has since the days of Diderot been seen as a condition of progress. Recent years have witnessed a felt need to communicate the cardinal principles of the modern understanding of the brain to the general public. Periodical articles designed to this end have become commonplace and books intended to acquaint the layman with the essentials of neuroscience are finding their way into libraries and stores.[13] These texts tend to use exuberant language to communicate the scope and promise of these discoveries to the reader. One example of this genre in a British newspaper informs the reader that the cerebral cortex is "Home to your humanity."[14] Another

---

[12] Presidential Proclamation 6158.

[13] The modernism and fixation with technology of some of this literature is startling. According to one text, "As we enter the twenty-first century functional brain scanning machines are opening up the territory of the mind just as the first ocean-going ships once opened up the globe. The challenge of mapping this world—locating the precise brain activity that creates specific experiences and behavioural responses—is currently engaging some of the finest scientists in the world." Rita Carter, *Mapping the Mind* (London: Weidenfeld & Nicolson, 1998), p. 6. As we have seen, the metaphor of brain-mapping and the image of the scientist as bold explorer is far from new.

[14] "It Makes You Think," *The Independent Magazine*, 31 October 1998, p. 94. One token of the presence of these forms of knowledge in popular culture are the parodies of the genre that sometimes appear. An article by Michael Rubiner in *The New York Times Magazine* of 30 April 1995 has, for instance, given its own wry comment on the supposedly mappable faculties of the modern American cerebral cortex. A reasonably faithful brain profile is accompanied by text listing a variety of localized functions at particular sites. Under the cate-

declares that modern neuroscience "is of immense practical and social importance because it paves the way for us to recreate ourselves mentally in a way that has previously been described only in science fiction." Thanks to these imminent technologies, "the individual's state of mind (and thus behaviour) will be almost entirely malleable."[15] Although a nod is made in the direction of the "ethical" questions that such power will raise, what is remarkable is the sheer enthusiasm that such prospects seem to invoke.

Visual representations of the brain figure prominently in such pieces. Typically, a human head is shown in profile with a section removed to expose the brain. Lines connect sections of the cerebrum to blocks of text that explain its functional significance. This style of representation harks back to the brain profiles developed in the nineteenth century by the pioneers of cerebral localization. Such illustrations are, however, increasingly supplemented by photographs that purport to show the brain actually at work; thanks to new technologies such as Positron Emission Topography, it is possible to show which parts of the brain "light up" when particular mental attributes are manifested. The implication is that these visualized phenomena are the true basis of those emotions or thoughts.

The enormity of the claims made for the modern brain are a justification for seeking to write its history. The theme of this book has been to reveal something of the contingencies attending the creation of the brain by means of literary and other forms of representation. Through these processes of writing and figuring the aphasic emerged as the bearer of the new brain and as a symbol of humanity's subjection to a mass of interwoven nerve cells. At the same time a template was formed for a new scientific endeavor dedicated to documenting the intricacies of that dependence. Within its own frame of reference this enterprise has been an astonishing success—hence the exultation surrounding current expositions of neuroscience. This is, moreover, an endeavor without limit or term: no matter how much is discovered about the brain there will always be more to learn. One has to be impressed with the grandeur of the outcome of over a century of work; the brain is indeed the most complex object in the known universe. We should pause, however, before allowing that is engrosses the whole of the humanity that created it.

---

gory of "Language" (located near Broca's region) the following faculties appear: Nicknames, Smooth Talk, Puns, Making Introductions, Doing Accents, Thank-you Letters. The author has, thanks to the solicitude of a friend, in his possession a greetings card bearing a diagram illustrating the essential attributes of the "Politician's Brain" in which "Longing for Extracurricular Sex" is, in conformity with phrenological doctrine, located in the cerebellum.

[15] Carter, *Mapping*, pp. 6–7.

INDEX